Global Health, Global Health Education, and Infectious Disease: The New Millennium, Part I

Guest Editor

ANVAR VELJI, MD

INFECTIOUS DISEASE CLINICS OF NORTH AMERICA

www.id.theclinics.com

Consulting Editor
ROBERT C. MOELLERING Jr, MD

June 2011 • Volume 25 • Number 2

SAUNDERS an imprint of ELSEVIER, Inc.

W.B. SAUNDERS COMPANY
A Division of Elsevier Inc.
1600 John F. Kennedy Blvd., Suite 1800, Philadelphia, PA 19103-2899.
http://www.theclinics.com

INFECTIOUS DISEASE CLINICS OF NORTH AMERICA Volume 25, Number 2
June 2011 ISSN 0891–5520, ISBN-13: 978-1-4557-0463-7

Editor: Barbara Cohen-Kligerman
Developmental Editor: Teia Stone

Infectious Disease Clinics of North America (ISSN 0891–5520) is published in March, June, September, and December by Elsevier Inc., 360 Park Avenue South, New York, NY 10010-1710. Periodicals postage paid at New York, NY and additional mailing offices. Subscription prices are $251.00 per year for US individuals, $435.00 per year for US institutions, $124.00 per year for US students, $297.00 per year for Canadian individuals, $538.00 per year for Canadian institutions, $355.00 per year for international individuals, $538.00 per year for international institutions, and $171.00 per year for Canadian and international students. To receive student rate, orders must be accompained by name of affiliated institution, date of term, and the *signature* of program/residency coordinator on institution letterhead. Orders will be billed at individual rate until proof of status is received. Foreign air speed delivery is included in all *Clinics* subscription prices. All prices are subject to change without notice. **POSTMASTER**: Send address changes to *Infectious Disease Clinics of North America,* Elsevier Health Sciences Division, Subcription Customer Service, 3251 Riverport Lane, Maryland Heights, MO 63043. **Customer Service: 1-800-654-2452 (US). From outside of the US and Canada, call 1-314-447-8871. Fax: 1-314-447-8029. E-mail: JournalsCustomerService-usa@elsevier.com (print support) or JournalsOnlineSupport-usa@elsevier.com (online support).**

Infectious Disease Clinics of North America is also published in Spanish by Editorial Inter-MÅdica, Junin 917, 1er A 1113, Buenos Aires, Argentina.

Reprints. For copies of 100 or more, of articles in this publication, please contact the Commercial Reprints Department, Elsevier Inc., 360 Park Avenue South, New York, New York 10010-1710. Tel. (212) 633-3812, Fax: (212) 462-1935, E-mail: reprints@elsevier.com.

Infectious Disease Clinics of North America is covered in *MEDLINE/PubMed (Index Medicus), Current Contents/Clinical Medicine, Science Citation Alert, SCISEARCH,* and *Research Alert.*

Printed and bound by CPI Group (UK) Ltd, Croydon, CR0 4YY

Transferred to Digital Print 2011

Contributors

CONSULTING EDITOR

ROBERT C. MOELLERING Jr, MD
Shields Warren-Mallinckrodt Professor of Medical Research, Harvard Medical School; Department of Medicine, Beth Israel Deaconess Medical Center, Boston, Massachusetts

GUEST EDITOR

ANVAR VELJI, MD, FRCP(c), FACP, FIDSA
Chief of Infectious Disease, Department of Infectious Disease, Kaiser Permanente, South Sacramento, Sacramento, California; Co-Founder, Global Health Education Consortium (GHEC); Clinical Professor, Department of Infectious Disease, School of Medicine, University of California, Davis, California

AUTHORS

MUSHTAQ AHMED, MBBS, FRCS
Associate Dean of Medical Education, Faculty of Heath Sciences, The Aga Khan University Medical College, Nairobi, Kenya

GEORGE A.O. ALLEYNE, MD, FRCP
Director Emeritus, Pan American Health Organization, Washington, DC

MEGAN A.M. ARTHUR, MSc
Program Coordinator, Global Health Programs, Faculty of Medicine, McGill University, Montreal, Quebec, Canada

ALEX O. AWITI, PhD
Resident Ecologist, The Aga Khan University, Nairobi, Kenya

ROBERT BATTAT
Medical Student, Faculty of Medicine, McGill University, Montreal, Quebec, Canada

ROBERT C. BOLLINGER, MD, MPH
Professor of Infectious Diseases and International Health; Director, Center for Clinical Global Health Education, Johns Hopkins School of Medicine, Johns Hopkins University, Baltimore, Maryland

TIMOTHY F. BREWER, MD, MPH, FACP
Director, Global Health Programs; Associate Professor, Faculty of Medicine, McGill University, Montreal, Quebec, Canada

JOHN H. BRYANT, MD
Formerly Dean, Columbia University School of Public Health, New York, New York; Emeritus Professor of Community Health Sciences, Aga Khan University, Karachi, Pakistan; Senior Faculty Associate, Department of International Health, Johns Hopkins School of Public Health, Baltimore, Maryland

XOCHITL CASTAÑEDA, MA
Director, Health Initiative of the Americas, University of California at Berkeley, School of Public Health, Berkeley, California

LORD NIGEL CRISP, MA
The House of Lords, London, United Kingdom

CAREY FARQUHAR, MD, MPH
Associate Professor, Division of Allergy and Infectious Disease, Departments of Medicine and Epidemiology and Global Health, University of Washington, Seattle, Washington

EMILY FELT, MPP
Program Analyst, Health Initiative of the Americas, University of California at Berkeley, School of Public Health, Berkeley, California

AMITA GUPTA, MD, MHS
Assistant Professor of Infectious Diseases and International Health, Deputy Director, Center for Clinical Global Health Education, Johns Hopkins School of Medicine, Johns Hopkins University, Baltimore, Maryland

MOSES KAMYA, MBBS, MMed, MSc, PhD
Chair and Professor of Medicine, Department of Medicine, Faculty of Health Sciences, Makerere University, Kampala, Uganda

ELLY KATABIRA, MBBS, MMed, FRCP(Edin)
Professor of Medicine, Department of Medicine, Faculty of Health Sciences, Makerere University, Kampala, Uganda

JENNIFER KATES, MA, MPA
Vice President; Director, Global Health and HIV Policy, Kaiser Family Foundation, Washington, DC

REBECCA KATZ, PhD, MPH
Assistant Professor of Health Policy and Emergency Medicine, Department of Health Policy, The George Washington University, School of Public Health and Health Services, Washington, DC

PATRICK W. KELLEY, MD, DrPH
Director, Boards on Global Health and African Science Academy Development, Institute of Medicine, National Academies, Washington, DC

JANE MCKENZIE-WHITE, MAS
Managing Director, Center for Clinical Global Health Education, Johns Hopkins School of Medicine, Johns Hopkins University, Baltimore, Maryland

NEAL NATHANSON, MD
Associate Dean, Global Health Programs, School of Medicine, University of Pennsylvania, Philadelphia, Pennsylvania

ANDRÉ-JACQUES NEUSY, MD, DTM&H
Vice President, International Program, Global Health Education Consortium; Executive Director, Training for Health Equity Network, Baisy-Thy, Belgium

BJÖRG PÁLSDÓTTIR, MPA
Director, Program Development, Training for Health Equity Network, Baisy-Thy, Belgium

ALLAN RONALD, MD, FRCPC
Distinguished Professor Emeritus, Department of Medicine, University of Manitoba, Winnipeg, Manitoba, Canada; Department of Medicine, Makerere University, Kampala, Uganda

MAGDALENA RUIZ RUELAS, MPH
Special Programs Coordinator, Health Initiative of the Americas, University of California at Berkeley, School of Public Health, Berkeley, California

W. MICHAEL SCHELD, MD
Makerere University, Department of Medicine, Kampala, Uganda; Bayer-Gerald L. Mandell Professor of Internal Medicine and Neurosurgery, University of Virginia, Charlottesville, Virginia

MARC SCHENKER, MD, MPH
Director, Migration and Health Research Center; Professor, University of California Davis School of Medicine, University of California at Davis, Davis, California

NELSON SEWANKAMBO, MBBS, MMed, DLaws(Hon)
Principal, College of Health Sciences, Professor of Medicine, Department of Medicine, Faculty of Health Sciences, Makerere University, Kampala, Uganda

ANVAR VELJI, MD, FRCP(c), FACP, FIDSA
Chief of Infectious Disease, Department of Infectious Disease, Kaiser Permanente, South Sacramento, Sacramento, California; Co-Founder, Global Health Education Consortium (GHEC); Clinical Professor, Department of Infectious Disease, School of Medicine, University of California, Davis, California

CAMER W. VELLANI, MD, FRCP
Distinguished University Professor, The Aga Khan University, Karachi, Pakistan

Contents

Preface: Global Health, Global Health Education, and Infectious Disease: The New Millennium, Part I xiii

Anvar Velji

Global Health: The Twenty-First Century Global Health Priority Agenda 295

George A.O. Alleyne

Growth in global health interest in the past 20 years has been overwhelming and many universities throughout the world have created departments or institutes of global health. The essence of global health has to be promoting health equity globally. The global health agenda must embrace design of mixed health systems, involving both private and public components to address the emerging threat of noncommunicable diseases and existing communicable diseases as well as to reduce health inequity. The priority agenda for the twenty-first century is challenging but the improvements of the past give hope that the barriers to improving global health are surmountable.

Global Health: Evolving Meanings 299

Anvar Velji and John H. Bryant

Approaches to health, health care, and the terminology to describe global health have evolved over the past 70 years since the introduction of the Constitution of the World Health Organization and definition of health in broader terms. The early focus on individual care gradually shifted to community, population, and global approaches, with associated changes in the site of medical care, the personnel who provide it, and the education and training of those personnel. Concomitantly, goals changed from purely curative care to disease prevention and health promotion. Health was better understood to exist within the larger political, social, cultural, and ethical settings.

Global Health and the Role of Universities in the Twenty-First Century 311

John H. Bryant and Anvar Velji

A vast gap exists between knowledge, generation of knowledge, and the application of knowledge to the needs and benefit of the global population. In middle-income and lower-income countries, universities are becoming more engaged with the communities in which they are located to try to solve the difficult problems of poverty and poor health. Global collaborations and reform of medical education in the twenty-first century will help move universities out of cloistered academic settings and into the community to bring the changes needed to equitably meet the health needs of all.

Global Health Education Consortium: 20 Years of Leadership in Global Health and Global Health Education 323

Anvar Velji

The Global Health Education Consortium (GHEC) is a group of universities and institutions committed to improving the health and human rights of

underserved populations worldwide through improved education and training of the global health workforce. In the early 1990s, GHEC brought together many of the global health programs in North America to improve competencies and curricula in global health as well as to involve member institutions in health policy, development issues, and delivery of care in the inner cities, marginalized areas, and abroad.

Global Health: Networking Innovative Academic Institutions **337**

Björg Pálsdóttir and André-Jacques Neusy

Medically underserved communities suffer a high burden of morbidity and mortality, increasing with remoteness where access to health services is limited. Major challenges are the overall shortage and maldistribution of the health workforce. There is a lack of understanding of how academic institutions can best contribute to addressing these health inequities. A new international collaborative of health professions schools, Training for Health Equity Network, is developing and disseminating evidence, challenging assumptions, and developing tools that support health profession institutions striving to meet the health and health workforce needs of underserved communities.

Teaching the Basics: Core Competencies in Global Health **347**

Megan A.M. Arthur, Robert Battat, and Timothy F. Brewer

Compelling moral, ethical, professional, pedagogical, and economic imperatives support the integration of global health topics within medical school curriculum. Although the process of integrating global health into medical education is well underway at some medical schools, there remain substantial challenges to initiating global health training in others. As global health is a new field, faculties and schools may benefit from resources and guidance to develop global health modules and teaching materials. This article describes the Core Competencies project undertaken by the Global Health Education Consortium and the Association of Faculties of Medicine of Canada's Global Health Resource Group.

Global Health Capacity and Workforce Development: Turning the World Upside Down **359**

Lord Nigel Crisp

This article explores global health and the way in which the whole world is increasingly interdependent in terms of health. High-income countries need to help redress the balance of power and resources around the world, for self interest and self preservation if for no other reason. These countries have a particular responsibility to help support the training of more health workers and to strengthen health systems in low-income and middle-income countries. In this interdependent world, high-income countries can learn a great deal from poorer ones as well as vice versa, and concepts of mutuality and codevelopment will become increasingly important.

The Infectious Diseases Institute at Makerere University, Kampala, Uganda **369**

Allan Ronald, Moses Kamya, Elly Katabira, W. Michael Scheld, and Nelson Sewankambo

The Infectious Diseases Institute (IDI) at Makerere University, Kampala, Uganda, was created in 2001. This article outlines its origins, principles,

problems that may begin during transit and a number that occur as a result of migrants' socio-economic status in the receiving country. This article discusses the health status of Mexican immigrants in the United States including their access to health care, health disparities, and the social determinants of health among this population, with a focus on the health of women and children.

Global Health: Governance and Policy Development **435**

Patrick W. Kelley

Global health policy is now being influenced by an ever-increasing number of nonstate and non-intergovernmental actors to include influential foundations, multinational corporations, multi-sectoral partnerships, and civil society organizations. This article reviews how globalization is a key driver for the ongoing evolution of global health governance. It describes the massive increases in bilateral and multilateral investments in global health and it highlights the current global and US architecture for performing global health programs. The article closes describing some of the challenges and prospects that characterize global health governance today.

The Role of Treaties, Agreements, Conventions, and Other International Instruments in Global Health **455**

Jennifer Kates and Rebecca Katz

As nations become more reliant on each other for cohesive development of global health policies and practice, and globalization increasingly makes health challenges in one part of the world concerns for all nations, the importance and use of international agreements in framing policy and national commitments have increased. This article reviews international agreements, looking specifically at multilateral instruments or partnerships, to identify those that either directly focus on or encompass health. It defines the different types of agreements, describes the process through which governments enter into these agreements, evaluates the legality of agreements under international law, and assesses participation by member states.

Index **477**

FORTHCOMING ISSUES

September 2011

Global Health, Global Health Education, and Infectious Disease: The New Millennium, Part II
Anvar Velji, MD,
Guest Editor

December 2011

Biologic Response Modifiers in Infectious Diseases
Nancy Khardori, MD,
Guest Editor

March 2012

Device-Associated Infections
Preeti N. Malani, MD, MSJ,
Guest Editor

RECENT ISSUES

March 2011

Infection Prevention and Control in the Hospital
Keith S. Kaye, MD, MPH,
Guest Editor

December 2010

Diseases of the Gastrointestinal Tract and Associated Infections
Guy D. Eslick, PhD, MMedSC(Clin Epi), MMedStat, *Guest Editor*

September 2010

Emerging Respiratory Infections in the 21st Century
Alimuddin Zumla, FRCP, PhD(Lond), FRCPath, Wing-Wai Yew, MBBS, FRCP (Edinb), FCCP, and David SC Hui, MD(UNSW), FRACP, FRCP,
Guest Editors

ISSUES OF RELATED INTEREST

Clinics in Liver Disease February 2010 (Vol. 14, No. 1)
Health Care-Associated Transmission of Hepatitis B and C Viruses
Bandar Al Knawy, MD, *Guest Editor*
Available at: http://www.liver.theclinics.com/

Critical Care Clinics January 2011 (Vol. 27, No. 1)
Optimizing Antimicrobial Therapy of Life-Threatening Infection, Sepsis, and Septic Shock
Anand Kumar, MD, *Guest Editor*
Available at: http://www.criticalcare.theclinics.com/

Preface

Global Health, Global Health Education, and Infectious Disease: The New Millennium, Part I

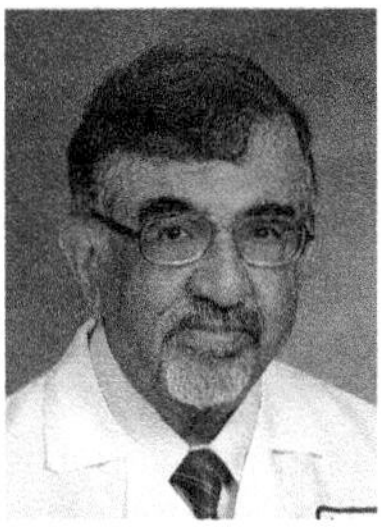

Anvar Velji, MD, FRCP(c), FIDSA
Guest Editor

DEFINING GLOBAL HEALTH AND ITS PARAMETERS

Attempts to define and draw the parameters of the newly emerging field of global health and global health education began over two decades ago. For instance, in 1990, over 22 global health experts contributed to the first volume on International Health in the *Infectious Disease Clinics*.[1] In 1995, 33 more experts contributed to the second volume on global health: International Health beyond the Year 2000.[2] The second volume drew this very insightful review:

> *"The collection of eye opening ideas contains more than visions. Thirty three excellent and expert authors have contributed 21 papers that embrace diversity of health concerns; not only with 1) basic biomedical and social sciences focused on major sets of health problems. There are papers that focus as well on 2) varied approaches to coping with health and developmental problems including ethical issues, information systems, anthropology and behavior changes and philosophy. It also addresses 3) educational approaches to the field of international health…I cannot expect to tell you about all the exciting ideas contained on these 225 pages…the volume also has articles which explore specific health concerns, including AIDS, major infectious diseases of Tropical Medicine, problems of systemic mycosis as infecting agents, diarrheal diseases, immunization successes, and women's health. Importantly, other articles tell the stories of advances in medical and health education, with examples of inter-institutional cooperation…"*[3]

The philosophical, ethical, and practical threads connecting these two foundational volumes of the *Infectious Disease Clinics* emerge from transformational visions and actions in global health, global health education, and the related disciplines of

Infect Dis Clin N Am 25 (2011) xiii–xxi
doi:10.1016/j.idc.2011.04.001

infectious disease, public health, and medicine in general. These ideas have been carried through the present issue and its companion, which will be published in September 2011.[4,5]

The new millennium opened with a focus on global equity, rights, social accountability, policies, and governance based on the principles of Health for All. These ideas, visions, and actions further consolidated various understandings and concepts of global health in an integrated world of information, knowledge, economies, trade, transport, risks, health, and health care products and services.

In the current issue of the *Clinics*, Sir George Alleyne, a past Director General of the Pan American Health Organization and recipient of the Global Health Education Consortium (GHEC) Distinguished Service Award in 1995, addresses three central issues in his editorial[6]: 1) the need for a widespread consensus on a working definition of global health, 2) the challenges of noncommunicable diseases, and 3) the need for competent health systems. The forthcoming high-level United Nations meeting in September 2011 will clearly elevate the importance of long-neglected chronic conditions and noncommunicable diseases.

Currently there is no worldwide consensus on a working definition of global health. In 2008, in Kampala, Nelson Sewankambo, the Principal of Makerere University, responded to my query very succinctly: "All we do in Africa, to us is global health." Suffice it to say that most authorities would agree that global health as a discipline and an area of study research and action refers to the health of all people at individual and population levels, with equity, universal access, affordability, and quality as hallmarks of such care.

TRANSFORMATION OF GLOBAL HEALTH EDUCATION IN THE 21ST CENTURY

The road to health equity in the 21st century is through transformation of education from prekindergarten, through primary and secondary schools, to university and allied professional schools. Here we include other schools involved in global health, such as schools of law, engineering, agriculture, veterinary, and social sciences. The last two decades have seen great movement and momentum in transforming education in the health professions globally as part of an effort toward global health workforce development and capacity building. These changes and suggestions for future directions have been captured by many of the articles in this issue *of Infectious Disease Clinics* and the one to be published in September. Two articles written by Jack Bryant and me open this issue. The first discusses global health meanings, traces the roots of global health over the last several decades, and offers several definitions of global health currently extant.[7] We follow this with an article on the role of universities in the context of the tremendous interest in global health throughout university campuses in North America, Europe, and Australia and in some countries in Central and South America, Africa, and Asia.[8] Clearly articulated mission and vision statements and social accountability are needed to calibrate this interest to benefit all parties and to train the current and next generation of the global health workforce. In another article, I examine how over the last two decades GHEC has exemplified networking among universities in North America and universities in the low- and middle-income countries for the common public good.[9]

Björg Pálsdóttir and André-Jacques Neusy explore how academic institutions can contribute to redressing misdistribution and shortages in the health workforce globally. The new international collaborative of medicine and health sciences with a socially accountable mandate, Training for Health Equity Network (THEnet), is collecting and disseminating evidence, challenging assumptions, and developing tools that support health profession institutions striving to meet the health and health workforce needs of underserved communities globally. The schools are unique but share common principles and strategies, starting from the involvement of the communities that they serve and extending to equity and evidence-based curriculum and training. In the foreseeable future, THEnet will have significant influence on the development of new accreditation standards, which will provide evidence of a medical school's impact on the public good.[10]

In the forthcoming issue of the *Infectious Disease Clinics*, Judith Calhoun, Harrison C. Spencer, and Pierre Buekens[11] address competencies for graduate global health education. There is an urgent need to focus on competencies, uniform standards, and interprofessional education beyond silos. The authors provide an overview of competency-based education (CBE) and its impact in the United States today. Of great significance, the Association of Schools of Public Health Initiative focused on CBE and the development of a standardized global health competency model targeted at master's level students majoring in global health. The authors also provide recommendations addressing potential future trends and barriers to acceptance of CBE to help the many educators and trainers who are just embarking on the competency journey. Acceptance by professional organizations, accrediting bodies, and school-wide leadership are critical for wider diffusion and success of the program and for the development of an adaptable and productive workforce for global health and well-being.[11]

Megan Arthur, Robert Battat, and Timothy Brewer explore the emerging field of core competencies in global health for medical students. The recommendations were developed by a joint committee of GHEC and the Canadian Association of Faculties of Medicine Resource Group on Global Health. The authors present compelling arguments as to moral, ethical, professional, pedagogical, and economic imperatives in support of the integration of global health topics within medical school curricula.[12] Clearly the disproportionate global burden of disease, socio-economic determinants of health, migration, and population displacement, changing global environment, economics, politics, and governance need to be viewed through the lens of equity, human rights, ethics, social justice, and social accountability. The core competencies in undergraduate medicine and in postgraduate public health recommended by Arthur, Battat, and Brewer and Calhoun and Buekens set a new benchmark and foundation in transforming global health education. The students, residents, and young faculty are clearly invested in their own education; for example, they recently released *Global Health Training in Graduate Medical Education: A Guidebook*, published in conjunction with GHEC.[13]

GLOBAL HEALTH CAPACITY AND WORKFORCE DEVELOPMENT

Lord Nigel Crisp shares his vast experience and insight on global health capacity and workforce development. In his influential book *Turning the World Upside Down: The Search for Global Health in the 21st Century*, Crisp shatters many myths of innovation and development. New ideas, approaches, and practices to deal with some of the most pressing situations, such as HIV-AIDS, have come from middle- and low-income countries. Interdependence, mutuality of learning, co-development, and new ideas about service delivery and professional education are ushering in a new way of looking at the world of health. In this article, Crisp picks up on these core ideas and develops them further.[14]

Allan Ronald and colleagues contribute a fascinating history of the founding of a unique institution in Uganda, the Infectious Disease Institute (IDI). For 15 years, the late Merle Sande—past president of the Infectious Disease Society of America, a master teacher, clinician researcher, and friend—made a point to be in Sacramento for his "Merle Sande Hour Lecture" at the Annual Infectious Disease Symposium that I co-directed for a number of years. Many a time we discussed global health, and I felt he had a lot to contribute to that field. In 2000, he saw a perfect opportunity following the International AIDS Society Conference in South Africa and in 2003 launched the Academic Alliance for AIDS Care and Prevention in Africa (now the Accordia Foundation), a collaborative of sustained partnership using the principles and expertise of private sector entrepreneurs along with the science and capacity-building energy of academicians. The IDI is a truly remarkable organization; it is a partnership between an academic institution—Makerere University—represented by Nelson Sewankambo and David Serwadda; Pfizer, represented by Hank McKinnell, a former CEO; and other infectious disease colleagues from both North America and Uganda. The institute has successfully harnessed support from other academic institutions and pharmaceutical foundations. For example, since 2006, Baylor University, with financial support from Bristol-Meyers Squibb, has taken responsibility for the pediatrics and adolescent programs. The Gilead Sciences Sewankambo Scholar Program was designed in 2007 to be an extension of postdoctoral clinical training. The Joint Uganda Malaria Program (JUMP) was launched in 2007 with funding from Exxon Mobile and the leadership of Moses Kamya and colleagues from the University of California, San Francisco.[15] The recent Institute of Medicine committee that produced the report "Preparing for the Future of HIV/AIDS in Africa: A Shared Responsibility" was co-chaired by Tom Quinn from Johns Hopkins and David Serwadda from Makerere. The report recommends that both the United States and individual African nations develop 10-year strategic "roadmaps" for combating AIDS, and that these prioritize prevention. It also urges long-term capacity building to produce the institutions and health workforce in Africa equipped to tackle the epidemic. Africa continues to face great challenges, and Africans should increasingly take up ownership of their health and well-being.[16] I firmly believe that IDI will be at the forefront of such efforts. It is clear from the IDI experience that the pharmaceutical, vaccine, biologicals, and device industries and philanthropic foundations can work constructively for the betterment of the public good. Further examples of such collaborations are given in the article by Patrick Kelley in this issue,[17] described in more detail below.

Robert Bollinger, Jane McKenzie-White, and Amita Gupta share the lessons learned from the Hopkins Center for Clinical Global Health Education. How does an institution build a global health education network for both clinical care and research using innovative distance learning tools to reach the health care providers in the most remote and resource-limited communities? Synchronous and asynchronous communication tools today connect global communities for joint learning and teaching, as well as for classical one-to-one teaching. Synchronous learning platforms and formats use fiber and wireless networks that support use of e-mail, web streaming, video conferencing, chat rooms, social networks, cell phones, and smart devices. Asynchronous platforms include e-mail, on-line forums, and social networking sites. The e-connectivity has empowered south-south and north-south collaboration. A fascinating example given by the authors is the Raki Health Science Program in Uganda. Their seminal research on male circumcision and reduction of HIV acquisition risk, as well as their training of health workers in performing circumcision, has greatly decreased HIV-AIDS–related morbidity and mortality.[18]

Carey Farquhar, Neal Nathanson, and the Afya Bora Consortium Working Group focus on an African–U.S. partnership to train leaders in global health. The Consortium is developing a Global Health Leadership Fellowship for medical, nursing, and public health professionals, largely drawn from the four African partner countries Kenya,

Tanzania, Uganda, and Botswana. The primary purpose of the fellowship is to provide trainees with practical skills that will prepare them for future positions leading the design, implementation, and evaluation of large, high-impact programs in governmental agencies, nongovernmental organizations, and academic health institutions in their own countries.[19]

Mushtaq Ahmed, Camer Vellani, and Alex Awiti address the two-fold logistical challenge of implementing an integrated primary health care system and a novel medical education model in sub-Saharan Africa. The Aga Khan University (AKU) and the Aga Khan Development Network currently operate with admirable success in several countries among diverse cultures and mostly in unforgiving political, geographic, and socio-economic terrain. Two decades ago as visiting faculty in Karachi, I had a firsthand opportunity to observe how the community health workers, medical and nursing students, and physicians from AKU worked with the social workers from the communities of Baba Island, the Katchi Abadi settlements, and the primary care facilities in Hyderabad. AKU was then in the process of integrating the secondary and tertiary centers with the help and involvement of the government of the province of Sindh. In 2008, while I was in Nairobi at the AKU, Dean Ahmed and his colleagues briefed me on their fascinating long-term plans for the university campus in Arusha, Tanzania, which will focus on basic sciences and humanities and be linked to the medical and nursing school in Nairobi. As Ahmed, Vellani, and Awiti state, consideration of factors influencing human health and development must encompass all life stages, from fetus to adult. Likewise, universal primary education, including education for girls, is the key for future well-being and health of societies. The authors also point out the need for a coordinated multi-sectoral approach to the sustainable development of integrated primary care, with the involvement of ministries and civil societies.[20]

Xochitl Castañeda, Magdalena Ruiz Ruelas, Emily Felt, and Marc Schenker address the health of migrants and the challenges they face, such as health threats, violence, and lack of human rights. The authors, who have a long and rich experience in migrant health, suggest that current work and future energies should be focused in a new direction, that of social determinants of health of these marginalized populations globally, rather than just focusing on prevalent infectious diseases and chronic noncommunicable diseases and their treatment. Intergenerational poverty, lack of education, jobs, housing, and health security are critical factors that need to be addressed if these populations are not to be viewed as minorities or others and are to be brought into the mainstream.[21]

Patrick Kelley from the Institute of Medicine brings his valuable experience to focus on governance and policy development in a rapidly changing global health landscape. Collective global action is increasingly being recognized as central to achieving the highest attainable standards of health and well-being for the world's people. A collaborative approach to implementation depends on carefully crafted, coordinated policies, for example, the landmark 2003 WHO Framework Convention on Tobacco Control[22] and the 2005 revision of International Health Regulations.[23] Kelley reviews the current architecture of global health governance and future challenges through the lenses of the functions and actions of world agencies, philanthropic organizations, public-private partnerships, and the role of civil societies.[17] The recent events in the Middle East and North Africa demonstrated the power of civil societies and social networks. If this type of power was harnessed for global health, education, and societal good in general, there would be acceleration in achieving the Millennium Development Goals and other, future, goals of creating a fair, socially just society.

Jennifer Kates and Rebecca Katz discuss the role of treaties, agreements, conventions, and other international instruments in global health.[24] In a broad review, the authors identify 50 international health agreements, including the International Sanitary Convention, which marked the first international health agreement of its kind. The authors discuss these agreements by type and focus and whether they are binding or nonbinding. The HIV-AIDS pandemic and several other infectious diseases have underscored the importance of such agreements for the global public good. This review also addresses how such health agreements underpin policy formulations and global health diplomacy as we move to addressing more complex global issues, such as gender discrimination, tobacco control, environmental issues, and other formidable challenges.

CONCLUSION

As C.E. Winslow remarked, "the life of the physical body is brief; but the thoughts of [human beings] have acquired immortality through the magic of the pen and of the printing press...a striking example of the miracle of the written word."[25] This may be equally applicable to all the experts and leaders in global health that have been assembled for these volumes and who today are marking out a new era and traveling the uncharted waters with knowledge and a moral compass to improve health for all human beings. When the history of global health and global health education is written, our experts' vision and generosity will be much appreciated, as they took on the grandest challenges in public health the Health for All. Global health, in short, will be all about how to advance equity in the 21st century.

The next volume in this series[5] will open with an editorial (by this author) on the transformation of global health, global health education, infectious disease, and chronic conditions and will continue with contributions on the landmark model for global health and global health education in the 21st century. Haile Debas and Thomas Coates of the University of California Global Health Institute explore the opportunities and challenges of setting up a center of excellence in global health. Julio Frenk, Octavio Gomez-Dantes, and Felicia M. Knaul make significant contributions to our understanding of global health by addressing the rapidly evolving challenges to health presented by rapid globalization, with a focus on infectious disease. Marcella M. Alsan, Michael Westerhaus, Michael Herce, Koji Nakashima, and Paul E. Farmer focus on the relationship of poverty, global health, and infectious diseases using their extensive experience from Haiti and Rawanda, where the Partners in Health has had a deep commitment and involvement for many years. Tracey Koehlmoos, Shahela Anwar, and Alejandro Cravioto focus on the neglected and severely neglected diseases and emerging issues such as climate change from their long, valuable experiences in Bangladesh. Nisha Garg focuses on neglected diseases and access to medicines through the five-pronged approach articulated by the WHO. Robert Martin and Scott Barnhart expertly address the long-neglected aspects of global laboratory systems development, with a particular focus on sub-Saharan Africa. Hadley Herbert, Adnan Hyder, and Alexander Butchart discuss one of the most neglected areas of global health: that of injury and violence, which rank among the ten leading causes of death worldwide. Ilona Kickbusch and Paulo Buss address the emerging important discipline of global health diplomacy and its application to peace and health. Cordelia Coltart, Mary Black, and Phillipa Easterbrook discuss the long tradition and involvement of the United Kingdom and its universities in global health, a wonderful addition to the discussion by Nigel Crisp in the current volume. Walter Patrick, a leader in global health for over two decades, shares his observations and perspectives on networking using the example of the Academic Consortia and Partnerships for Health in the Asia Pacific Region. Joel G. Breman, Kenneth Bridbord, Linda E. Kupfer, and Roger I. Glass discuss in great detail the historical, current, and future role of the Fogarty International

Center of the National Institutes of Health in training the global health workforce in the fields of infectious and chronic conditions; and Rossana Peeling and Solomon Nwako bring a fresh perspective on the complex issues of diagnostics research and drug innovations and applications to global health in the new millennium.

Previous volumes of the *Clinics* on Global Health were dedicated to great leaders in global health, such as Halfden Mahler, MD, of WHO, who led the Health for All Movement; His Highness the Aga Khan, whose health, development, education, and resource programs dot some of the most unforgiving terrain in the world; Mother Theresa, who worked in the slums of Calcutta and inspired so many; and "globalists" such as Carl Taylor, MD, Jack Bryant, MD, and Victor Neufeld, MD.

In keeping with that spirit, this volume is dedicated to Haile Debas, MD, a friend and fellow African, who is currently the Executive Director of the UCSF Global Health Sciences, Director of the UC Global Health Institute, and Chair of the Consortium of Universities for Global Health. Dr Debas established the Bellagio Essential Surgery Group (a consortium of 12 African countries, the WHO, and universities in the US and Europe), and the partnerships between UCSF and the Muhibili University Allied Health Sciences in Dar es Salaam, Tanzania. The Professor Haile Debas Centre for Health Professions Education at Muhibili University was inaugurated in his honor. He has co-chaired the Committee on Antiretroviral Drug Use in Resource-Constrained Settings, Board on Global Health, and is author of the report *Scaling Up Treatment for the Global AIDS Pandemic: Challenges and Opportunities* published by the committee. He chaired the Biological Sciences and Engineering Committee at the African Institute of Science and Technology of the Nelson Mandela Institution. In addition, he serves on several advisory committees to the Institute of Medicine and NIH. Recently he led UCSF in the signing of the Memorandum of Understanding with The Aga Khan University and serves as a trustee on its Board. His vision transcends boundaries, and that has facilitated the founding of the Global Health Institute at UCSF that serves the 10 UC campuses and co-ordinates their activities in several arenas of global health. Haile above all is a wonderful human being.

Last but not least we wish to thank Dr Robert Moellering, a leader in both clinical and investigative aspects of infectious disease and the Consulting Editor of the *Infectious Disease Clinics of North America*, for inviting me again to bring together the current influential opinion makers in global health, global health education, infectious disease, and public health. We also wish to convey our sincerest thanks to Barbara Cohen-Kligerman and all her staff for the excellent and timely help and wisdom they provided to me and the other authors.

ACKNOWLEDGMENTS

This work was supported by funding from Kaiser Permanente. The author wishes to thank Naomi L. Ruff, PhD, ELS, for copyediting assistance.

Anvar Velji, MD, FRCP(c), FIDSA
Department of Infectious Disease, Kaiser Permanente
South Sacramento
6600 Bruceville Road
Sacramento, CA 95823, USA

E-mail address:
Anvarali.Velji@kp.org

REFERENCES

1. Velji AM. International health. Infect Dis Clin North Am 1991;5(2).
2. Velji AM. International health, beyond the year 2000. Infect Dis Clin North Am 1995;9(2).
3. Markwardt R. Book review: International health beyond the year 2000. Leadership Public Health 2000;5(2):34–5.
4. Velji A. Global health, global health education, and infectious disease: the new millennium, Part I. Infect Dis Clin North Am 2011;25(2), in press.
5. Velji A. Global health, global health education, and infectious disease: the new millennium, Part II. Infect Dis Clin North Am 2011;25(3), in press.
6. Alleyne A. Global health: the twenty-first century global health priority agenda. Infect Dis Clin North Am 2011;25(2), in press.
7. Velji A, Bryant J. Global health: evolving meanings. Infect Dis Clin North Am 2011; 25(2), in press.
8. Bryant J, Velji A. Global health and the role of universities in the twenty-first century. Infect Dis Clin North Am 2011;25(2), in press.
9. Velji AM. Global Health Education Consortium: 20 years of leadership in global health and global health education. Infect Dis Clin North Am 2011; 25(2), in press.
10. Pálsdóttir B, Neusy A. Global health: networking innovative academic institutions. Infect Dis Clin North Am 2011;25(2), in press.
11. Calhoun J, Spencer HC, Buekens P. Competencies for global health graduate education. Infect Dis Clin North Am 2011;25(3), in press.
12. Arthur AM, Battat R, Brewer R. Teaching the basics: core competencies in global health. Infect Dis Clin North Am 2011, in press.
13. Chase J, Evert J, editors. Global health training in graduate medical education: a guidebook. 2nd edition. San Francisco (CA): Global Health Education Consortium; 2011. Available at: http://globalhealtheducation.org/resources/Documents/Both%20Students%20And%20Faculty/GH_Training_in_GME_Guidebook_2Ed.pdf. 2011.
14. Crisp N. Global health capacity and workforce development: turning the world upside down. Infect Dis Clin North Am 2011;25(2), in press.
15. Ronald A, Kamya M, Katabira E, et al. The Infectious Diseases Institute at Makerere University, Kampala, Uganda. Infect Dis Clin North Am 2011;25(2), in press.
16. The Great Beyond. Institute of Medicine urges ramp-up of AIDS prevention in Africa—November 29, 2010 [blog]. Available at: http://blogs.nature.com/news/thegreatbeyond/2010/11/institute_of_medicine_urges_ra.html.
17. Kelley P. Global health: governance and policy development. Infect Dis Clin North Am 2011;25(2), in press.
18. Bollinger R, McKenzie-White J, Gupta A. Building a global health education network for clinical care and research. The benefits and challenges of distance learning tools. Lessons learned from the Hopkins Center for Clinical Global Health Education. Infect Dis Clin North Am 2011;25(2), in press.
19. Farquhar C, Nathanson N. The Afya Bora Consortium: an African-US partnership to train leaders in global health. Infect Dis Clin North Am 2011;25(2), in press.
20. Ahmed M, Vellani C, Awiti A. Medical education: meeting the challenges of implementing primary health care in sub-Saharan Africa. Infect Dis Clin North Am 2011;25(2), in press.
21. Castañeda X, Ruiz R, Felt E, et al. Health of migrants: working towards a better future. Infect Dis Clin North Am 2011;25(2), in press.

22. World Health Organization. WHO framework convention on tobacco control. Available at: http://whqlibdoc.who.int/publications/2003/9241591013.pdf.
23. World Health Organization. International health regulations (2005). Geneva (Switzerland): World Health Organization; 2008. Available at: http://www.who.int/ihr/9789241596664/en/index.html.
24. Kates J, Katz R. The role of treaties, agreements, conventions and other international instruments in global health. Infect Dis Clin North Am 2011;25(2), in press.
25. Winslow CE. The message of Lemuel Shattuck for 1948. Am J Public Health Nations Health 1949;39(2):156–62.

Global Health: The Twenty-First Century Global Health Priority Agenda

George A.O. Alleyne, MD, FRCP

KEYWORDS

• Health • Global • Chronic diseases • Inequity

The growth in global health interest in the past 20 years has been overwhelming. There is strong academic interest with many universities in the developed and developing world, creating departments or institutes of global health, and the growth in writing on this subject is perhaps well exemplified by the fact that the title "global health" generates 275 million items in Google. The philanthropic attention to global health problems has been well manifested in the Bill and Melinda Gates Grand Challenges in Global Health, which has identified 14 major health challenges in the developing world and seeks to develop technologies to address them.[1] Thus, in one sense, the priorities at least for research have been identified.

But there are other facets of global health that occupy the attention of the world in the twenty-first century. This issue of *Infectious Disease Clinics* demonstrates the numerous aspects of global health and the number of existing health problems that can be addressed under this rubric. However, the author contends that major conceptual issues as well as thematic health concerns remain and they will be embraced by the workers in this field as part of the agenda for the twenty-first century, attracting attention and hopefully, funding.

There are 2 aspects that the author wishes to address briefly. First, there needs to be more widespread consensus on a working definition of global health, because unless there is some common understanding, it will be difficult to measure progress. The difficulty of consensus is shown, for example, by the recent affirmation of the European Commission, "Global health is a term for which no single definition exists."[2] This difficulty is in spite of the major effort of Koplan and colleagues[3] to develop a definition based on a careful analysis of the antecedents of global health, tracing the origins through public health and international health. Sometimes the author was concerned that in some quarters, global health is nothing more than international health in

The author has nothing to disclose.

Pan American Health Organization, 525 Twenty-Third Street, NW, Washington, DC 20037, USA
E-mail address: alleyned@paho.org

Infect Dis Clin N Am 25 (2011) 295–297
doi:10.1016/j.idc.2011.02.009 **id.theclinics.com**

new wineskins and much of that international health was not international sensu stricto but really attention to the health of the developing world by practitioners from the developed world without any reference to the role of nations or national entities, which is obviously implied in the term international.

The first part of the definition given by Koplan and colleagues[3] reads "global health is an area for study, research and practice that places priority on improving health and achieving equity in health for all people worldwide." The definition stresses the health of all people and not the health of only the developing world and emphasizes what to the author is the essence of global health practice, the reduction of disparities, and the search for more health equity globally. The new agenda should address the fundamental question as to whether this quest for equity is intrasocietal or intersocietal. Most of the emphasis on the social determinants of health and the possibility of addressing them relate to the inequalities within the state or society where there is a responsible government that can and should reduce the inequities that occur. In economic terms, there is theoretically an agent responsible to the principals, the members of that society, for actions to redress the inequities. But if there is indeed to be global health, meaning the health of all people regardless of national domicile, then attention must be paid to the disparities between countries or societies and the current lack of an identifiable agent to remedy the situation if indeed a whole global society can be cast in the role of principal. The answer will probably come from the establishment of some form of health governance completely different from the existing arrangements that give priority to governments. Daniels[4] frames the issue in terms of the possibility of egalitarianism being able to exist outside of a society within which there are formal relational arrangements.

The thematic priorities for the twenty-first century for global health depend essentially on 2 factors: (1) the burden of disease and the application of appropriate instruments to reduce it and (2) the degree of inequality that exists for these diseases within and between countries or societies. In terms of the burden of disease, the new phenomena are the growing importance of the chronic noncommunicable diseases (NCDs) and the erosion of the difference in addressing these compared with the traditional communicable or infectious diseases. It is, of course, clear that more and more of the NCDs are being shown to be infectious in origin, and with improvements in therapy, more of the communicable diseases will need chronic care. With appropriate therapy, AIDS is rapidly becoming a chronic illness.

At present, the NCDs represent the largest cause of death globally, and the major NCDs cardiovascular disease, cancer, diabetes, and chronic respiratory disease are projected to account for 41 million deaths worldwide in 2015.[5] Remarkably, these diseases were not included among the Millennium Development Goals (MDGs), and the presumption was they were essentially diseases of the rich and the elderly and did not represent the degree of inequity that was manifested by the major infectious diseases. In addition, the advent of human immunodeficiency virus infection and the successful advocacy for it as a developmental issue obscured the problem of chronic diseases to some extent. It has been recognized in the review of the MDGs in September 2010 that the NCDs are important and there is now good evidence of the significant economic burden they impose and that the world will not achieve the MDGs unless attention is paid to the NCDs as well.[6] Many of the myths surrounding these diseases are being dispelled; for example, the aging phenomenon plays a minor role in the mortality of these diseases as compared with the effect of social and economic conditions.[7] The importance of these diseases has been recognized internationally to the extent that the United Nations will convene a High Level Meeting in September 2011 with the participation of Heads of State and Government, specifically to address the problem of chronic diseases.[8] The outcome of this meeting will inform the priority agenda in this area for the foreseeable future.

It is counterproductive to pit one set of diseases against another, and instead the emphasis must be on the appropriate technologies and interventions and the health systems to apply them. The NCDs share some common risk factors that are modifiable through changes of individual personal behavior coupled with government action to so modify the enabling environment to make the healthy choice the easy one. These risk factors include tobacco use; diet, particularly the excess use of salt; and lack of physical activity.

The global agenda to address the relevant priority health needs must embrace the design of systems that are mixed in most part of the developing world, involving both public and private components.[9] There are many facets to health system design, and the World Health Organization Framework for Action represents a good synthesis of the important elements.[10] The Framework's 6 building blocks for an efficient system are all important, but according to the author, the aspect of health financing and the provision of universal access to services is the one that speaks more to reducing the inequity that is so central to global health. Countries will apply different recipes, but the essential elements must be that the burden of the cost of health care is shared among the population more widely, the threat of health care–induced poverty is removed, resources are better used, and the health outcomes are better.

The priority agenda for the twenty-first century is obviously a daunting one, but the improvements of the past give hope that the barriers for achieving the global health equity are not insurmountable.

REFERENCES

1. Varmus H, Klausner R, Zerhouni E, et al. Grand challenges in global health. Science 2003;302:398–9.
2. European Commission. The EU role in global health. Communication from the Commission to the Council, the European Parliament, the European Economic and Social Committee and the Committee of the Regions. Brussels (Belgium): European Commission; 2010. 31.3.2010 COM (2010) 128 final.
3. Koplan J, Bond TC, Merson M, et al. Towards a common definition of global health. Lancet 2009;373:1993–5.
4. Daniels N. International health Inequalities and global Justice. In: Boylan M, editor. International public health policy and ethics. Dordrecht (The Netherlands): Springer; 2009. p. 109–30.
5. Strong K, Mathers C, Leeder S, et al. Preventing chronic diseases: how many lives can we save? Lancet 2005;366:1578–82.
6. Stuckler D, Basu S, McKee M. Drivers of inequality in millennium development goal progress: a statistical analysis. PLoS Med 2010;7(3):e1000231.
7. Stuckler D. Population causes and consequences of leading chronic diseases: a comparative analysis of prevailing explanations. Milbank Q 2008;86:273–326.
8. United Nations. Prevention and control of non-communicable diseases. New York (NY): United Nations ; 2010. Resolution A/64/L.52.
9. Nishtar S. The mixed health system syndrome. Bull World Health Organ 2010;88: 74–5.
10. World Health Organization. Everybody's business: strengthening health systems to improve health outcomes. WHO's Framework for Action. Geneva (Switzerland): WHO; 2007. ISBN 978 92 4 159607.

Global Health: Evolving Meanings

Anvar Velji, MD, FRCP(c), FIDSA[a,b,*], John H. Bryant, MD[c,d]

KEYWORDS

- International health • Geographic medicine
- New (transitional) international health • Global health
- What is global health? • Definition(s) of global health
- Global health human rights • Global health ethics

HISTORICAL ROOTS OF GLOBAL HEALTH

Over the past six to seven decades there has been dramatic progress globally in ideas, ideals, and values about how health is viewed beyond healthy lifestyles to well-being and a clear moral commitment to equity and rights in provision of health care. The World Health Organization's (WHO's) goal of Health for All (HFA) by the year 2000, announced in 1978,[1] was a truly remarkable and unprecedented effort to harness technologic capacities and political forces to social purpose on a global scale. This was a radical break with the past, introducing values, structure, and function different from those that previously governed health and the health care sector and applying them not only to health services but also to the workforce and education at universities and schools of public health.[2] These changes included rights and social reforms pertaining specifically to health. The future of public health would never be the same, and the authors believe that these dramatic forces mark the beginning of global health. The HFA movement acquired considerable legitimacy and support when it was ratified by 160 member countries of the WHO that supported its values and principles. These were later translated into health policies by member states. The three identified components—health service, workforce, and higher education—continue to underpin major global health policies.[3]

This work was supported by funding from Kaiser Permanente.
[a] Department of Infectious Disease, Kaiser Permanente, 6600 Bruceville Road, South Sacramento, CA 95823, USA
[b] Department of Infectious Disease, School of Medicine, University of California, Davis, CA, USA
[c] Department of International Health, Johns Hopkins School of Public Health, Baltimore, MD, USA
[d] Columbia University School of Public Health, Emeritus Professor of Community Health Sciences, Aga Khan University, Karachi, Pakistan
* Corresponding author. Department of Infectious Disease, Kaiser Permanente, 6600 Bruceville Road, South Sacramento, CA 95823.
E-mail address: Anvarali.Velji@kp.org

Infect Dis Clin N Am 25 (2011) 299–309
doi:10.1016/j.idc.2011.02.004 **id.theclinics.com**

HFA was not simply an extension of previous values, structures, and function. The roots of HFA were in the social, technical, and political trends that had affected thinking about health care in both less developed and more developed countries. These trends set the stage for HFA, the Millennium Development Goals (MDGs), and global health. These powerful trends are briefly outlined.

Justice and Equity

Justice and equity acquired a prominent and insistent role beyond lip service and thus became embedded in social systems,including health. This meant delivery of effective services must be continually paired with access.[4]

Changing Ideas on the Nature of Development

New styles of development were sought that were rooted in human values and that connected social and economic aspects of development. Overdependency on donor countries began to be transformed into self-sufficiency.

Roles of Communities and the Society

Members of the community, and for that matter the larger society, now had an insistent voice and could effectively express their concerns and be active participants in decision making over passive participation. Trends in the health sector were developing in parallel to social changes. There was an increased awareness that overemphasis on curative medicine (the biologic model) not only was detrimental but also had a distorting effect on health services; an increasing realization of the importance of disease prevention and health promotion; evolution of the concept of primary health care (PHC), including community-oriented PHC; and changing views on the health workforce, including the emergence of various alternatives to physician-centered care.

These trends initially emerged slowly but rapidly gathered intensity and are now at hurricane strength with the arrival on the world stage of global health, which encompasses and draws together many of the concepts of social, technical, political, and ethical thought.[5] The major components of HFA—health services, health workforce, and higher education—continue to be stressed in the MDGs and in global health (discussed by Bryant and Velji elsewhere in this issue).[6,7]

The first and foremost elements of PHC, as defined in WHO's Health For All Meeting at Alma Ata, now known as Almaty, Kazakhsatan,[8] are education concerning prevailing health problems and methods of prevention and control; promotion and provision of adequate food supply and appropriate nutrition; adequate supply of safe water and basic sanitation; maternal and child health, including family planning; immunization against the major infectious diseases; prevention and control of locally endemic diseases; appropriate treatment of common diseases and injuries; and provision of essential drugs. Thus, it is intended that PHC should be developed so as to ensure that that there is universal coverage. The services provided under this coverage should be relevant, effective, acceptable, and affordable and should cover the full range of preventive, curative, and rehabilitative activities. The services should further involve communities so as to promote self-reliance and lessen dependencies and should integrate health and development generally.[9]

EVOLUTION TO GLOBAL HEALTH

The authors have identified four periods of time that mark major changes in the ways the three components of the health sector have been defined in their objectives, functions, and capabilities: the individual health era, the community health era, the population health era, and the global health era (**Table 1**).

The Individual Health Era

Before World War II, health care focused primarily on the treatment of the individual. Curative care reigned supreme. There were also major advances in public health that benefited all countries. This era was both the individual health era as well as the physician-centered era, and the services were mostly provided in hospitals, health centers, and physician offices. Nurses and auxiliaries were seen as aides to assist the physician rather than to provide care on their own.

The Community Health Era

After World War II, more attention was given to extending health services to larger populations, with increased emphasis on public health and preventive programs. In the workforce sector, there was a shift towards nonphysicians fulfilling some tasks previously done by physicians. A two-tier system evolved. At one level, doctors and nurses provided care at a hospital or major health center; at a second level, a group of auxiliaries staffed a network of health centers or dispensaries, providing care in the facilities and through mobile teams to surrounding communities. The major shortcoming was the lack of health workers and budget; coverage, therefore, could only be extended to 10% to 20% of rural populations. There have been examples of such services reaching every household, however, such as auxiliaries keeping records of services, with special concern for the well-being of young children.

The Population Health Era

The foremost goal of health services in relation to HFA is explicitly universal PHC coverage, and the key concept on which universal coverage is built is the demographically defined population. A second goal, which assumes great importance in the long term, is that PHC be both relevant and effective with respect to the current and emerging health problems of the population. In developing countries, where equity of access is still a distant hope and quality care is available to few, the overriding priority is generally coverage with PHC while still trying to maintain relevance and effectiveness.

The Global Health Era

Between the years 1989 and 1996, many disciplines came together to focus on global health problems. This period can be designated as the dusk of international health and the dawn of global health. The dusk-dawn metaphor represents gradual and overlapping changes in understanding, articulation, and actions in achieving equity and health for all, as well as in the creative education of health professionals to solve the countless problems of ill health tied to the political, social, and economic forces of globalization. For instance, the landmark *Infectious Disease Clinics of North America* issues on international health (global health) in 1991 and 1995[10,11] were devoted not only to defining the problems of the new broader concepts of global health, such as an aging population; maternal, infant, and childhood morbidity and mortality; AIDS and other infectious diseases; chronic conditions; drug and nicotine addiction; and environmental deterioration, but also to health systems, limited resource availability, and the close relationship between health and education. The most significant issues then and now, however, are poverty and marginalization of girls and women. Here are two quotations by His Highness the Aga Khan IV, who founded the first university

Table 1
Evolving approaches to health services, workforce, and higher education

Era	Coverage	Health System	Workforce	Education
Individual health	Individuals	Hospitals Health centers	Doctors, assisted by nurses and auxiliaries	Clinical
Community health	Selected aspects of communities	Hospitals Health centers Selected communities and components of PHC	Doctors Nurses Auxiliaries	Prevention Social factors Roles of team in PHC
Population health (HFA)	Universal, with effective services	Defined populations Total coverage PHC to communities Community participation Relation to development	Doctors Nurses Auxiliaries Community level workers	Competencies for universal coverage Human resource development Relation to socioeconomic development
Global health (HFA, MDGs, human rights, ethics, governance)	Individual, community, and global populations	Global Centers of Excellence Health systems built on the bedrock of equity, access, affordability, and quality	Team concept	Global perspectives on patterns of disease Social cohesion Pursuit of equity

Data from Bryant JH. Health services, health manpower, and universities in relation to health for all: an historical and future perspective. Am J Public Health 1984;74(7):714–9.

based on the principals of HFA, in Karachi, Pakistan. The first quotation relates to poverty and the urgency to address it:

There are those who enter the world in such poverty that they are deprived of both the means and the motivation to improve their lot. Unless they can be touched with the spark which ignites the spirit of individual enterprise and determination, they will sink into apathy, degradation, and despair. It is for us who are more fortunate to provide that spark.[12]

The second quotation relates to the persistent marginalization of women:

Just as health care and medical education are critical beacons in the struggle of a community to achieve its highest potential, the status of women and the professions they serve are decisive criteria. They cannot be realized without the full participation and leadership of qualified and creative women. The way that the community or a nation excludes or enables women to fulfill its most vital tasks bespeaks its failure or success. There is neither democracy nor meritocracy in a society that excludes half its members.[12]

DEFINING HEALTH

Prior to defining global health and its several dimensions, it is important to acknowledge the most useful and pervasive definition of health, which is written into the constitution of the WHO and has not changed since 1946: "Health is a state of complete physical, mental and social well-being and not merely the absence of disease or infirmity."[13]

The Ottawa Charter for Health Promotion[14] emphasized the concept of health promotion, which it defined as a process of enabling people to increase control over, and to improve, their health. To reach a state of complete physical, mental, and social well-being, an individual or group must be able to identify and to realize aspirations to satisfy needs and to change or cope with the environment. Health is seen as a resource for everyday life. Therefore, health promotion not only is the responsibility of the health sector but also goes beyond healthy lifestyles to well-being. The charter went on to identify the fundamental conditions and resources necessary for health, such as peace, shelter, education, food, income, a stable ecosystem, sustainable resources, and social justice and equity. Good health was seen as a major resource for social, economic, and personal development and an important dimension of quality of life. Furthermore, because health can be influenced by multiple factors, such as political, economic, social, cultural, environmental, behavioral, and biologic factors, health promotion advocacy was emphasized.[14] Promotion of health equity focuses on the central tenet of HFA. Equity is defined as "ensuring equal opportunities and resources to enable all people to achieve their fullest health potential." The charter went further and included a secure foundation in a supportive environment, access to information, life skills, and opportunities for making healthy choices.[14] The charter emphasized that people could not achieve their fullest health potential unless they were able to take control of those factors that determine their health.[14]

INTERNATIONAL HEALTH, GEOGRAPHIC MEDICINE, AND THE NEW (TRANSITIONAL) INTERNATIONAL HEALTH

International Health

In the early 1980s, one definition of international health focused on health activities between governments or people from two or more nations, thus including WHO disease control programs, clinical services provided by medical missions and corporations, overseas research by universities, and populations and nutrition activities associated with health programs.[15] The author of the *Textbook of International Health* offered this definition: "[International Health] is a systemic comparison of the factors that affect the health of all human beings," and then wryly added, "Please feel free to write your own definition. It is a big subject that can accommodate many interpretations."[16] International health lends itself to both reductionist and integrative paradigms. For one of the authors of this article (AV), the medical–public health approach to the definition led to the inclusion of multiple disciplines of public health, tropical medicine, geographic medicine, infectious diseases, nutrition, maternal and child health, aging, and other areas of concern, all falling under the rubric of the broader term, *international health*, that is akin to the global health paradigm today. This broader concept of international health was about the health and welfare of global beings, no matter where they reside, and it had a second dimension of redesigning health systems to optimize health care delivery.[17]

Geographic Medicine

In the United States, there was an earlier attempt to widen the parameters of international health. Geographic medicine was seen as a new movement within international health and international medicine, and the divisions were located within the schools of medicine. This represented a top-down strategy whereas the other part of international medicine, PHC, was seen as a grass-roots effort to improve health that drew its strength from community-based projects, a variety of social sciences, health education, and the use of paramedical personnel. PHC needed tools, however, that geographic medicine could supply. Both efforts were directed to diseases of the developing nations. Geographic medicine was "created to encompass something exciting in the world of international health…[It] has brought diseases of the developing nations into the mainstream of medical science."[18] These two approaches were thought to offer complementary solutions to the problems of the developing nations.

The New (Transitional) International Health

Parallel attempts to widen the definition and reach of international health were also taking place in the public health community in Mexico. Frenk and Chacon[19] at the National Institute of Public Health in Cuernavaca, Mexico, proposed the concept of a "new international health." In contrast to the traditional international health, the new international health was based on the changing paradigms and shifts in relationships between societies globally and encompassed social, political, economical, and other forces. The need for this new approach had also been stated by others.[17]

This new or transitional international health was designed to respond to the interests of all countries, thus avoiding interpretations associated with a specific group of nations (referring to North America and Europe) and called for exchange of knowledge, ideas, and experiences among both developed and developing nations as well as training to solve health problems beyond boundaries.[19] This new international health recognized that economic, political, and social diversity is present in all countries, although problems and populations are specific within each subgroup. The new view recognized that the reality of global health problems is the responsibility of all; many unsolved health problems are shared between all countries regardless of their development status and require collaboration and cooperation of all in their solutions;

there is an essential need for cooperation in training, research, and sharing of knowledge.

Frenk and Chacon[19] saw the new international health as having three aspects: (1) a field of knowledge, (2) a field of enquiry, and (3) an arena for action. The new international health defined public health by the distinctive feature of analysis at the population level, with populations represented by components of the international community, such as nations with cultural and territorial identity; states, as the political organization of nations; entities, comprising multiple nations, such as economic, political, and military blocs; and international organizations, whether public, private, for profit, or nonprofit. Furthermore, as a field of enquiry, it was conceived as the interdisciplinary study of health phenomena as they occur among the members of the international community. It addresses the effects of economic, political, and social forces that transcend boundaries, their relations and effect on health, and the reciprocal effect of health on those forces. As an arena for action, this new international health is the systematic effort to identify health conditions and to organize health responses among and by the subjects of the international community. Thus, it includes international policy making and technical cooperation to characterize health needs and to mobilize resources in order to respond to those needs.[19]

Focusing on training human resources, generation of knowledge, and the practice of international health, Frenk and Chacon[19] pointed out that the focus on health conditions and health systems extended beyond boundaries. Because public health provides the theoretic, methodologic, and technical elements to approach the study of the outcomes of specific populations, problems, and programs and brings together disciplines, such as epidemiology, demography, economics, sociology, administrative sciences, law, and ethics, the combination of public health and the new international health could consolidate the field and enrich public health. A new concept of international health with a vigorous intellectual and academic tradition would support the generation of knowledge and its application.

DEFINING GLOBAL HEALTH

There are multiple expressions of global health in the international literature, and it is useful to review selected examples, because they call attention to diverse dimensions of global health. Without exposure to such examples, perspectives can remain limited in this rapidly evolving field. Some representative samples of statements on global health have been selected from diverse sources to highlight the discussion.

Global Health in Transition: A Synthesis: Perspectives from International Organizations, 1996

The reports reviewed and the ideas presented in *Global Health in Transition* signaled a world of great and accelerating change whose effects pervaded the fields of health and social development.

> *The paradox—one we tentatively view with hope—is that, amidst volatility and frustration, and partly because of them, consensus has evolved nonetheless and in some generally common directions: toward fuller comprehension of the hard demands of development, the potential of more effective methods for coping with its obstacles, and more awareness about the larger global context in which development must be addressed.*[20]
>
> *[G]iven the complexity of the problems, the certainty of uncertainty, the urgency for allocating all manner of resources more wisely, the rapidity of movements of people and information—separation from collective action makes scant sense.*

Indeed, it is difficult to imagine significant advances...without a truly interactive global community honestly, modestly, and realistically engaged in the further elaboration and pursuit of the Next Agenda in Global Health.[20]

From Julio Frenk's Address at the Harvard School of Public Health Commencement, June 7, 2007

More today than ever, global health is in need of a renewed ethic, the ethic of universal rights, so that every human being may have an opportunity to achieve his or her full potential. These are the fundamental values that have nourished public health, both as a field of inquiry and as an arena for action...." [Actions are guided by] "...two powerful sources of illumination—ideas and ideals. Ideas take the form of knowledge derived from science. Ideals take the form of values derived from ethics. Ideas can be transforming to the evidence base for sound decision-making. Ideals can be transformed into the integrity base for coherent action.[21]

The Expert Committee on the U.S. Commitment to Global Health, Convened by the Institute of Medicine, National Academy of Sciences, 2008

Global health is the goal of improving health for all people in all nations by promoting wellness and eliminating avoidable disease, disabilities, and deaths. It can be attained by combining population-based health promotion and disease prevention measures with individual-level clinical care. This ambitious endeavor calls for an understanding of health determinants, practices, and solutions, as well as basic and applied research on risk factors, disease, and disability.[22]

Alma-Mata: Definition of Global Health, March 2009

Global Health is a field of practice, research, and education focused on health and the social, economic, political, and cultural forces that shape it across the world. The discipline has an historical association with the distinct needs of resource-poor countries but it is also concerned with health-related issues that transcend national boundaries and the differential impacts of globalization. It is a cross-disciplinary field, blending perspectives from the natural and social sciences and the humanities to understand the social relationships, biological processes, and technologies that contribute to the improvement of health worldwide.[23]

Jeffrey Koplan and Colleagues: "Towards a Common Definition of Global Health," 2009

A steady evolution of philosophy, attitude, and practice has led to the increased use of the term global health. Thus, on the basis of this analysis, we offer the following definition: global health is an area for study, research, and practice that places a priority on improving health and achieving equity in health for all people worldwide. Global health emphasizes transnational health issues, determinants, and solutions; involves many disciplines within and beyond the health sciences and promotes interdisciplinary collaboration; and is a synthesis of population-based prevention with individual-level clinical care.[24]

Nigel Crisp: Turning the World Upside Down

"My perspective of global health is terribly simple. I use the term...to embrace all those health issues that affect us all, rich and poor." (Lord Nigel Crisp, MA, personal communication, February 3, 2010). Crisp identifies these issues as (1) shared vulnerability to epidemics of diseases that can affect economies, international relationships, and health; (2) interdependence in terms of international regulations; setting of standards from disease prevention to professional practice and sharing of medical records; standard definitions of health professions; shared knowledge, workforce, pharmaceuticals, and vaccines; and shared assumptions and behaviors; and (3) recognition of economics and international relationships. "Like swine flu, the credit crunch swept around the world very rapidly, after a long incubation in the excesses of the [19]90s and early 2000s" (Lord Nigel Crisp, MA, personal communication, February 3, 2010).

In addition to the preceding definitions and understandings of global health, the authors have used the shared ideas, ideals, and values in their definition of global health to emphasize the notions of equity, justice, fairness, rights, solidarity, compassion, and mutual respect: global health is a new paradigmatic vision and action that rests on human ideas, ideals, and values of providing high quality of health for all globally. It has at its core equity, compassion, altruism, sharing, sensitivity, dignity, respect, philanthropy, and professionalism. It is bound by a global ethical code of conduct and governance that transcends borders, ethnicity, caste, and religions. It enshrines the notion of the global good. Global health as a collective entity and enterprise is beyond the component disciplines, philosophies, and sciences but is informed by them. As a new mindset, global health is mindful of individual liberties and societal good. It enshrines the principles of equity, solidarity, beneficence, avoidance of malfeasance, promotion of fairness, and autonomy with responsibility. Global health is mindful of the privileged connections that exist between all human beings. It is science based and evidence based and is informed by socially sensitive input of all parties involved.

CHALLENGES IN DEFINING GLOBAL HEALTH

The authors believe that, although global health as an emerging discipline increasingly seems to be a single definable entity, it is made up of many complex ideas, ideals, and actions that have shifting and fluid boundaries. Global health as a collective entity has sociophilosophic and moral dimensions that are often neglected in the quest for defining the discipline of global health. The bellwether of societal good is the good of the individual, which the authors have called the global being. It is the individual good that bespeaks and reflects the good of the communities, societies, and nations. One of the authors of this article (AV) stated that "good global health" is delivering the promise of health for all in an equitable manner.[9] In practical terms, these powerful ethical actions have been used successfully by Frenk and colleagues[25] to launch the landmark Mexican health reforms on a bedrock of ethics, values, empathy, rights, equity, evidence-based interventions, and science. Focusing on another aspect of global health action, that of philanthropy, William Foege at the Gates Foundation stated unequivocally, "global health is about caring about unnecessary suffering, the premature death, and the unmet potential in the world...applications of tools, resources in correcting these problems...it is about noticing and caring about blatant unfairness...it is about not ignoring acute problems like famine."[26]

For the authors, the concept of global health reaches beyond the rich-poor dichotomy and geographic boundaries and borders to the forces that separate the powerful, free, privileged populations from the population that is powerless and unfree. In its acceptance of human diversity, global health is an expression of support for the human rights enshrined in the WHO constitution, charters, and declarations and in the instruments of governance of several other nation-states.

SUMMARY

The rich diversity of views expressed and the discussion in this article emphasize the necessity of a broad definition of global health based on global health ethics and practical disciplinary approaches to equity, human rights, and evidence-based interventions and actions. The examples given illustrate that these principles are becoming the cornerstones in the educational institutions involved in global health and within the matrix of philanthropy in general as well as public health policy. The authors expect that the recent increased collaborations between the schools of public health and medicine in the unifying field of global health will result in increasing the number of global health leaders and developing a competent health workforce. It will rapidly eradicate the barriers between universities and schools of public health globally. Multidisciplinary and transdisciplinary approaches in solving the diverse health, research, service, development, and environmental issues are bringing forth novel collaborations across agriculture, veterinary sciences, engineering, politics, civic societies, ethics, and law. These collaborations between the countries of the north and south and between south and south continue to be strengthened as there is a new-felt urgency of sharing and solving problems together.

ACKNOWLEDGMENTS

The authors wish to thank Naomi L. Ruff, PhD, ELS, for reviewing the manuscript and for her helpful suggestions and assistance with copyediting.

REFERENCES

1. World Health Organization. Declaration of Alma-Ata. Alma-Ata, USSR 1978. Available at: www.who.int/hpr/NPH/docs/declaration_almaata.pdf. Accessed November 22, 2010.
2. Bryant JH. Health services, health manpower, and universities in relation to health for all: an historical and future perspective. Am J Public Health 1984;74(7):714–9.
3. Frenk J. Keynote address, human rights and global health: the case of a successful reform. Paper presented at: 17th Annual GHEC Conference: global health ethics and human rights: practical applications to multicultural health. Sacramento (CA), April 16, 2008.
4. Bryant JH. Principles of justice as a basis for conceptualizing a health care system. Int J Health Serv 1977;7(4):707–39.
5. Velji A, Bryant JH. Global health ethics. In: Markle W, Fisher M, Smego R, editors. Understanding global health. Columbus (OH): McGraw Hill; 2007. p. 295–317.
6. Bryant JH, Velji AM. Global health and the role of universities in the twenty-first century. Infect Dis Clin North Am 2011;25(2), in press.
7. Velji A. Global Health Education Consortium: 20 years of leadership in global health and global health education. Infect Dis Clin North Am 2011;25(2), in press.
8. World Health Organization. Global strategy for health for all by the year 2000. Geneva (Switzerland): World Health Organization; 1981.
9. Velji A. International health. West J Med 1991;155(3):308–9.
10. Velji AM, editor. International health. Beyond the year 2000. Infect Dis Clin North Am 1991;5(2):183–436.
11. Velji AM, editor. International health, beyond the year 2000. Infect Dis Clin North Am 1995;9(2):223–461.
12. Velji AM. Preface. Infect Dis Clin North Am 1991;5(2).
13. World Health Organization. Constitution of the World Health Organization. Available at: http://apps.who.int/gb/bd/PDF/bd47/EN/constitution-en.pdf. Accessed June 15, 2010.

14. World Health Organization. Ottawa charter for health promotion. First International Conference on Health Promotion. 1986. Ontario (Canada). Available at: http://www.who.int/hpr/NPH/docs/ottawa_charter_hp.pdf. Accessed April 11, 2010.
15. Baker TD, Weisman C, Piwoz E. United States health professionals in international health work. Am J Public Health 1984;74(5):438–41.
16. Basch PF. Textbook of international health. New York: Oxford University Press; 1999.
17. Velji AM. International health. Beyond the year 2000. Infect Dis Clin North Am 1991;5(2):417–28.
18. Olds GR. Geographic medicine: a new movement within international health. Acad Med 1989;64(4):190–2.
19. Frenk J, Chacon F. International health in transition. Asia Pac J Public Health 1991;5(2):170–5.
20. Bryant JH, Harrison PF. Global health in transition: a synthesis: perspectives from international organizations. Washington, DC: National Academy Press; 1996.
21. Frenk J. 84th commencement address, Harvard School of Public Health. Available at: http://harvardmagazine.com/commencement/public-health-commencement-address. Accessed July 28, 2009.
22. Institute of Medicine Committee on the U. S. Commitment to Global Health. The U.S. commitment to global health: recommendations for the public and private sectors. Washington, DC: National Academies Press; 2009. Available at: http://www.nap.edu/catalog.php?record_id=12642. Accessed April 11, 2010.
23. Alma Mata. Alma Mata proposal for postgraduate medical training in global health. Executive summary. Available at: http://www.almamata.net/news/system/files/Postgraduate%2520training%2520in%2520Global%2520Health%2520Proposal.pdf. Accessed June 30, 2010.
24. Koplan JP, Bond TC, Merson MH, et al. Towards a common definition of global health. Lancet 2009;373(9679):1993–5.
25. Frenk J, González-Pier E, Gómez-Dantés O, et al. Comprehensive reform to improve health system performance in Mexico. Lancet 2006;368(9546):1524–34.
26. McCarthy M. A conversation with the leaders of the Gates Foundation's Global Health Program: Gordon Perkin and William Foege. Lancet 2000;356(9224):153–5.

Global Health and the Role of Universities in the Twenty-First Century

John H. Bryant, MD[a], Anvar Velji, MD, FRCP(c), FIDSA[b,c,*]

KEYWORDS

- Universities and global health • Equity • Global collaboration
- Advocacy • Education reforms
- Socially accountable education • Social determinants of health
- Health systems • Capacity building

The new millennium has ushered in an era of rapid transformation, affecting socioeconomic, environmental, cultural, financial, political, and academic arenas globally across societies that are now closely intertwined.[1] The generation of knowledge and its optimal use and application, especially in the field of global health and development, have garnered significant attention in recent years. Universities play a vital role as generators and guardians of education, research, service, advocacy, and policy development and ideally are expected to act in concert with society as new challenges and opportunities emerge.

Universities have classically followed four forms of scholarship: the scholarship of discovery (research); the scholarship of integration (making connections across disciplines); the scholarship of application (using scholarship to solve problems); and the scholarship of teaching (transmitting, transforming, and extending knowledge).[2] To this is added the scholarship of policy development, diplomacy, and advocacy. Today, with the demands of globalization and the rapid generation and transmittal of knowledge, as well as goods, services, infections, chronic conditions, and harmful behaviors, universities are increasingly becoming active institutional agents of change in many spheres beyond their traditional calling.

This work was supported by funding from Kaiser Permanente.

[a] Department of International Health, Johns Hopkins School of Public Health, Baltimore, MD, USA

[b] Department of Infectious Disease, Kaiser Permanente, South Sacramento, 6600 Bruceville Road, Sacramento, CA 95823, USA

[c] Department of Infectious Disease, School of Medicine, University of California, Davis, CA, USA

* Corresponding author. Department of Infectious Disease, Kaiser Permanente, South Sacramento, 6600 Bruceville Road, Sacramento, CA 95823.

E-mail address: Anvarali.Velji@kp.org

Infect Dis Clin N Am 25 (2011) 311–321

doi:10.1016/j.idc.2011.02.012

id.theclinics.com

Changes in academic perspectives have a special value in developing economies where new universities are being established to deal with the nearly intractable problems of development. The burdens of development are multiple, varied, and complex, and the response of universities can be substantial in selected areas to which they have given priority. Several institutions have embarked on an interdisciplinary approach to addressing the problems of poverty, equity, and societal marginalization and their negative consequences. With this widened scope, universities are being called on to provide practical solutions to these problems by working at the intersections of policy, trade, and health with education, health development, diplomacy, agriculture, veterinary applications, engineering, and social sciences.

This article highlights how universities have addressed the major challenges of the past century and the first decade of the twenty-first century as they transition from a biologic model of medicine to a new paradigm of global health. This dramatic change has its roots in the Health for All movement, which articulated several core principles. The authors believe that the global health movement is a successor of that call and is based on the principles of equity, fairness, and justice and thus has the power to bridge the century-old schism between medicine and public health.[3]

The role of universities in middle-income and lower-income countries in health systems development has always been challenging because they often operate amidst economic crises and uncertainties as well as civil and political unrest. Furthermore, they depend on unpredictable foreign aid. Despite this setting, universities see it as one of their prime missions to bring about certainty and stability to the extent possible. A classic question facing universities is whether they should remain in the academic cloister, protecting their independence and stability yet risking relevance to societal need, or venture out to grapple with the problems of society and prove their capacity for dealing with the world around them, even though this might put their independence and stability at risk. In practice, experience ranges from gingerly putting an academic toe in the societal waters of a community to becoming extensively involved in the development of the health systems at a national level.[4] This article examines several avenues that universities have pursued to get involved with global health problems despite myriad challenges.

UNIVERSITIES AND GLOBAL HEALTH: VISION AND MISSION STATEMENTS

Academic values and societal concerns often guide the mission and vision of universities and their academic health centers. Medical schools, the most powerful and often the most prestigious part of a university due to large budgets and considerable independence, have repeatedly been criticized for abrogating their responsibility and social contract with the public. The mission and vision of some schools, however, such as the Aga Khan University in Karachi, Pakistan, stands in stark contrast to the status quo. The original mission statement was revised to state that its education, research, and service are oriented toward improving the health of the people of Pakistan and the developing world and the health services that serve them. This statement focuses on improving health rather than providing health care and on improving health services rather than accepting the notion that health services are only the responsibility of the government. The mission statement is put into practice by the objectives and the actions of Aga Khan University's Department of Community Health Sciences, which emphasizes the development of health systems in Pakistan through education, research, and development of health systems prototypes in collaboration with local and national authorities as well as educating health personnel for leadership positions.[5]

Thus, mission statements play a critical role in directing the vision of institutions seriously contemplating involvement on global health (see the article by Palsdottir and Nuesy elsewhere in this issue, which discusses Training for Health Equity Network schools, for an example[6]).

UNIVERSITIES AND GLOBAL HEALTH: REFORM OF MEDICAL EDUCATION

Over the past several decades, there have been countless conferences, articles, and learned reports with suggestions for how to reform medical education and for how medical schools should train future doctors to focus on populations as well as individual care. A century after the original reforms initiated by Abraham Flexner and the Carnegie Foundation,[7] a new paradigm for medical education is long overdue. These reforms, introduced in the first decade of the twentieth century, had three major components: inclusion of all medical schools within universities, a robust basic science curriculum, and the use of university hospitals for clinical instruction and teaching as well as for imposing stricter oversight and criteria for admission. What has often been overlooked are Flexner's other relevant suggestions that physicians display humility and focus on preventive aspects rather than purely curative aspects of care and his view that medical schools are public service corporations and thus are socially accountable.[8]

Academic health centers in the United States and Canada have long been recognized as key components of universities and premier scientific and technical repositories. They have also been credited for dramatic responses to complicated, individual-centered care in the latter half of the twentieth century. Other medical issues, however, such as chronic conditions, aging, equity in care, and escalating costs in the face of poor health indices in the population, have largely been neglected. This pattern was also copied in the middle-income and lower-income countries that adopted the Western academic center paradigm. To change the status quo, Health of the Public: An Academic Challenge, was founded in 1986 by The Pew Charitable Trusts and the Rockefeller Foundation to help academic health centers adapt to changes in demographics and the health care environment. A new mission statement was created and launched. By 1992, 17 Health of the Public institutions in the United States had implemented 7 major objectives of the mission[9]:

1. To provide basic competencies in population health to all health professional students. Students were to learn basic concepts in epidemiology, psychology, sociology, biostatistics, ethics, health economics, and family dynamics. Teaching was to be interdisciplinary, involving both medical and nonmedical fields, and was to occur within the health center and in community centers.
2. To provide joint degrees in medicine and public health for those who wished to pursue population health.
3. To provide preventive care and care that promotes health rather than just curative care.
4. To conduct research in population medicine using multidisciplinary expertise, including epidemiology, behavioral sciences, economics, policy analysis, and clinical decision making.
5. To assume institutional responsibility for maximizing the health of a defined population.
6. To learn and develop expertise in development and deployment of health resources.
7. To provide sociopolitical advocacy for the health of the population.

UNIVERSITIES, HEALTH SYSTEMS, AND CAPACITY BUILDING

Neither approach, primary health care or disease-oriented intervention, alone has been successful in achieving the goals of global health, despite significant funding by governments and philanthropies. Since 2000, the focus has shifted to the development of efficient and responsive health systems. Here lie great opportunities for universities in developing health systems and building capacity. The World Health Organization defines health systems as including "all the activities whose primary purpose is to promote, restore, or maintain health."[10] The improvement and performance of health systems vary with each country's priorities, political and economic circumstances, social values, leadership at national levels, and the appropriate mix of the trained workforce to be commensurate with the needs of societies. Variables, such as the presence of multilateral partners, nongovernmental organization density, and activities of philanthropic groups with their own agendas, are substantial forces that may act negatively on fragile health systems. In contrast, civic society ownership and active participation are valuable attributes and often the hallmarks of successful systems. The challenge for universities participating in global health is how to help create and sustain robust health systems tailored to each community by evaluating what already exists, taking note of stakeholders, opinion leaders, and the availability of sustained resources in the milieu of the rapidly changing global health structures. Several models and strategies have been devised to strengthen health systems to achieve the Millennium Development Goals by 2015; despite the importance of these goals, several of them are unlikely to be met, especially in fragile states, such as those in sub-Saharan Africa.

In most African countries, health continues to be in crisis mode, with serious staffing and resource deficits. This has been especially true since 1989, the onset of the HIV/AIDS epidemic, with ongoing malaria, tuberculosis, other infectious diseases and chronic conditions, aging, postconflict displacement, and rampant poverty. This is compounded by the global economic crisis. In addition, gender disparities in education persist, and opportunities for minorities and women continue to lag. Fewer than 500 full-time senior health staff are available to provide care for more than 900 million people in Africa, and approximately two-thirds of them are male; more than half (55%) of countries do not have any postgraduate public health program.[11] Yet there is a new optimism growing about health and development in Africa as democratization of the continent increases and, most importantly, so does the clarity of the African voice and initiative for public health and its governance. The New Partnership for Africa's Development has called for increased public health education and training capacity in Africa.[12,13]

UNIVERSITIES IN MIDDLE-INCOME AND LOW-INCOME COUNTRIES

Universities in developing countries face a daunting task as they seek to develop amidst pervasive underdevelopment. They are located in a familiar landscape of scarcity and complexity, the most obvious components of which are widespread ill health, unchecked population growth, and inequitably distributed, largely ineffective health services. To this mix can be added political instability, poor governance, cycles of violence, economic stagnation and corruption, and habitual disregard for and exploitation of the poor, which all increase the difficulty in providing care in an equitable manner. Nevertheless, serious attempts are being made from which the universities in the developed world have often learned and benefited. For instance, between 1962 and 1984, a series of meetings was convened by medical schools in Dakar, Senegal; Ibadan, Nigeria; Kampala, Uganda; and Ouagadougou, Burkina Faso to examine the role of universities in health and development. The focus of the meetings was on how to foster the idea of implementing service through practical training and reconciliation of culture and tradition with the environment as well as understanding the political commitment to the national effort and develop the workforce.[14]

US UNIVERSITIES AND THEIR ROLE IN GLOBAL HEALTH

Increasingly, North American and European universities are getting involved with long-term commitments in capacity building and training human resources. These universities have significant resources to play a key role in reducing global health disparities and the diseases of poverty, specifically through increasing the training, research, and service capacity of educational institutions in low-income and middle-income countries.[15] Paradoxically, global efforts have enabled some universities to better understand themselves, to collaborate across disciplines within their own institutions, and to enhance education and health care in local communities.[16] Global health provides an opportunity for academic institutions to put aside their competitive tendencies and work collaboratively to address global health challenges.[17] These interuniversity collaborative efforts have been the defining element of the Global Health Education Consortium over the past two decades 1989.[18] Health programs are increasingly viewed within their social, economic, and developmental contexts, including activities in agriculture, education, gender empowerment, water sanitation, nutrition transportation, communications, and microloans for small-business development.[19] As pointed out by some, university participation in assisting developing countries usually occurs as an offer of specific expert skills of a specific university or medical center department. Examples include Tulane University's expertise in monitoring and evaluation, Columbia University's expertise in mother-to-child transmission, and Baylor University's expertise in the treatment of pediatric AIDS.[20]

Some examples that illustrate the diverse missions, interests, and avenues used by some North American universities are highlighted:

1. International health was established as a distinct academic discipline at Johns Hopkins University in 1961. Today, it is the largest and oldest department of international health in the world. There are 510 active global health research and service programs directed by 361 faculty and staff of the Hopkins schools of medicine, public health, nursing, and Jhpiego (a nongovernmental organization). These are located in 117 countries.[21]
2. In 2007, Duke University and the National University of Singapore jointly opened their medical school based on the American style of postbaccalaureate medical education. The aim and emphasis of this collaboration is to prepare physician scientists for academic careers, with plans for 20% of each class to complete a combined MD/PhD degree. The new medical school in Singapore will be an integral part of the national investment in biomedical sciences that includes the establishment of Biopolis, which houses a national biomedical research hub of public and private institutions.[22]
3. The human-animal-environmental health interface is one of the most critical challenges facing humankind today. The premier One Health Center at the University of California, Davis, is a collaborative effort of multiple disciplines working locally, nationally, and globally to attain optimal health for people, animals, and the environment. In 2009, the University launched a new initiative, PREDICT, in hopes of preventing future global pandemics with millions of deaths. The PREDICT global consortium partners include the Wildlife Conservation Society, Wildlife Trust, Global Viral Forecasting, and the Smithsonian Institution.

   One of the authors of this article (AV) was a member of the committee that submitted the successful proposal for the One Health Center as part of the University of

California Global Health Institute. The following quotation is from that proposal: "While the One Health approach is being praised and encouraged nationally and internationally, there is more dialog than action. We propose the first academic-based center to advance One Health research, education, and practice...the One Health Center will train leaders in a trans-disciplinary, action oriented approach to confront problems that affect human, animal, and ecosystems health in diverse settings around the world" (Jonna Mazet, DVM, PhD, Kathryn Dewey, PhD, Christian Sandrock, MD. Proposal for a University of California School of Global Health Center of Expertise, unpublished material). The One Health Center is part of the newly minted University of California Global Health Institute.[23]

4. In 1974, Case Western Reserve University established the first Geographic Medicine Division within the Department of Medicine at the University Hospitals in Cleveland, Ohio. This was a new movement within international health. Historically, the study of tropical diseases had been relegated to the schools of public health, outside the mainstream of medical science.[21] Geographic medicine brought diseases of the developing world into the mainstream of medical science.

   It was also felt by some that creating a university-wide program or institute with internal organization and commitment from a university as a whole could be a more effective way to organize diverse scientific disciplines, such as medicine, molecular biology, anthropology, biostatistics, nutrition, and political science, into a cohesive group.[21] Such a prototype university-wide geographic medicine program was developed at Brown University in 1987 under the umbrella of an international health institute; however, "it represented a 'top down' strategy. It was realized that alliances and partnerships would have to be forged with other major forces in international medicine such as primary health care, with their essentially 'bottom-up' or 'grass-roots' strategy."[21] Within the Global Health Education Consortium, in contrast, several family physicians, public health workers, medical specialists, program directors, and other educators, as well as students, continue to work closely for the betterment of global health, both in North America and abroad.

EUROPEAN UNIVERSITIES AND GLOBAL HEALTH

In the European Union, there is a renewed interest in developing world-class universities comparable to those in the United States to effect a successful transition to a knowledge-based economy and society. Although there are more than 4000 institutions of higher learning in Europe, the Commission of the European Communities felt that there was too much mediocrity and duplication and not enough of the critical mass necessary to support excellence.[24] Lambert and Butler wrote, "Too few of them are international centers of research excellence, attracting the best talent from around the world. Their efforts in both teaching and research are limited by a serious, and in many areas desperate, lack of resources."[25] Many of the universities, however, have had major impacts in tropical medicine and infectious disease research, education, and service. Now there are major efforts to accelerate their involvement in global health. Unfortunately, space prevents describing these efforts in detail in this article.

HOW CAN UNIVERSITIES ADDRESS THE SOCIAL DETERMINANTS OF HEALTH?

Education is a boon to individuals and is a public good. Universities have a central role to play in both aspects. Research shows that primary education is, globally, a route to better health for those who have it and for their children. Increasingly, it has been recognized that we must not stop there. Women with secondary education have children who are more likely to survive than women without secondary education. For those concerned about population growth, the answer appears to lie in education of women. Those with secondary education have fewer children than those with less education.

Data from high-income countries show that the apparent health benefits to education continue: people with university education have better health than those without. Although it has always been the case that not everyone can go to university—a source of inequality—it is likely that an increasing proportion going to university means that the health benefits are more widely shared.

But education is also a public good. Universities shape society through building knowledge and understanding of the world. Universities are the source of creative and critical thinking that advance every sphere of human activity, not least those factors that affect human health and well-being.

In addition to the contribution to knowledge and critical understanding of social trends, universities interact with the communities in which they are situated, the business community, and wider society, initiating and catalyzing both ideas and services, and driving innovation that contributes a substantial amount of present and future revenue to the national and global economy. Universities are also economic entities that provide employment to a sizeable and growing workforce; in England, for example, more than 314,000 people are employed in higher education.[26]

The Commission on Social Determinants of Health placed social justice, empowerment, and evidence at the heart of action to reduce health inequalities between and within countries. Empowerment of the individual, communities, and whole nations is fundamental to improving conditions that create health inequalities. Universities have a key role to play in the Commission's three dimensions of empowerment: material—meeting the material needs for a healthy life; psychosocial—enabling a sense of control over life; and political—voice and participation in decision-making processes. Evidence guides action on the social determinants of health through building understanding of both the causes of health inequalities and how to act effectively to tackle the causes of health inequalities.[27,28]

WHAT CAN UNIVERSITIES DO?

The current and ongoing challenge is for universities to get involved beyond their walls into societal problems under the rubric of social determinants of health. The authors offer the following recommendations:

1. The pursuit of global health challenges universities to go beyond the traditional boundaries and parameters of education, research, and service. Any cloistered university that still pursues global health without leaving the campus should transcend these walls and join the call of Health for All.
2. Global health centers and their universities in high-income countries should commit themselves to the pursuit of social justice, equity, and human rights by engaging the problems of society both locally and globally.
3. Universities should recognize that the resistant problems of health are embedded in poverty and other economic and sociocultural factors. Universities should try to minimize these hurdles while simultaneously advancing the health of the populations. They should build a science-based capacity for analyzing health in general and health systems, in particular. The analytic capacity should be focused on local problems, providing essential input to policymaking and program development. Universities should pursue the development of health services in relationship to

underdevelopment wherever they are located. Universities can explore the feasibility of achieving equity, effectiveness, efficiency, and quality of care in health services and can seek to develop effective links between health policy, diplomacy, management, monitoring, and evaluation.

4. Another major role that universities should undertake is in developing leadership. Preparing students to lead in global health and its related fields is critical. The curricula should reflect today's problems and those that are likely to be present in the next few decades. The relationship between university partnerships should go beyond mutual academic enrichment.
5. Universities should build partnerships with communities, because community involvement is not only a social and philosophic nicety but an imperative for development because it has power to shape millions of lives and improve productivity.[29]

The long-term relationship between Moi University in Eldoret, Kenya, and the University of Indiana in the United Sates is an example of how universities can work together in the interest of global health.

Several important outcomes have emerged from the Indiana–Moi partnership, such as several new facilities in Kenya that were made possible by private philanthropy (eg, operating theaters and a mother and baby hospital); postgraduate training programs in medicine and pediatrics; leadership development of Moi University faculty members and their engagement in national policy; the evolution of the Academic Model Providing Access to Healthcare consortium of North American partners; burgeoning research; 50 full-tuition scholarships that the University of Indiana makes available through the dean of the Moi University School of Medicine to support its most impoverished students; food and income security programs that touch the lives of more than 30,000 persons daily; a program that is reaching out to more than 10,000 orphans and vulnerable children; and the expansion of the academic partnership to schools of law, nursing, and liberal arts. The Indiana–Moi model consists of a continuous on-site presence of faculty members; an emphasis on the tripartite academic mission, but with a "care first and leave nobody behind" mindset; a foundation of individual counterpart relationships based on mutual respect and benefit; a population perspective (that is, an expectation that Indiana and Moi really are responsible for the health of the population); and a highly entrepreneurial mode with its expectation to create wealth (R.M. Einterz, MD, Indiana University, personal communication, September 27, 2010).

HISTORIC PERSPECTIVES ON THE ROLES OF UNIVERSITIES IN HEALTH—NATIONAL AND GLOBAL

In 1969, one of the authors of this article (JHB) wrote a book, *Health and the Developing World*,[30] that was the product of an extensive study sponsored by the Rockefeller Foundation. The study involved 2 years of visiting and studying 22 developing countries, guided by an oversight committee consisting of outstanding internationalists in the health sector.

Among the issues relating to international health was the dilemma faced by universities as to whether they would concentrate mainly on the promotion of academic excellence, defined in terms of high-quality medical care mainly within the walls of a university hospital, or, alternatively, concentrate on the health problems of the nation, which would be addressed through focusing on the needs of the people and their communities, which reached beyond hospital-based care to community-based care. The book concluded that this issue was of crucial importance for universities and should be addressed in ways that would seek an effective and balanced involvement in both options.

Moving ahead into the current century, it can be asked, How relevant are those questions to the current context of university function? It is fair to say that similar questions are still priorities but need to be extended to the global level. Thus, a major change in the challenges to universities seen over these 40 years is the extension from national to global considerations. Also, the capacities for universities to address the important issues of health and development, given the scope and complexity of those issues, have grown substantially.

SUMMARY

Reflecting on the roles of universities in relation to global health in 2011 and 1969,[30] there is a vast gap that continues to exist between biomedical knowledge and the capability of bringing this knowledge within effective reach of the world's people. Whether or not that gap is narrowed and the rate at which it is narrowed depend on the development of an appropriate health workforce that is commensurate with the needs of the population, efficient agencies for delivering health care, robust health systems, political will, societal involvement and ownership, social responsiveness and accountability of the educational institutions, and philanthropic alignment to development and health priorities determined by the local populations.

As the year 2015 is approached, the great unmet health need, the serious deficiencies in health care systems, and the most telling educational inadequacies cluster around the single but painfully complex question of how to provide care for large numbers of people with limited resources. A special burden rests on universities, for there resides the potential for defining the necessary directions for change and for educating the leadership that can bring those changes to reality. The changes that are needed call for new phases of technologic development, new forms of professional capability, new relationships among health personnel, new approaches to educational problems, and new attitudes of professionals and those in academia. Because the most fundamental purposes of universities are involved, it must be asked how those purposes can be changed. There is a need to look again at the concept of excellence and the meanings universities attach to it. The authors see a dilemma. If universities turn away from involvement in the community in favor of pursuing scholarship within their own walls, its scholarly successes will only distantly benefit the nation and its people. If, alternatively, universities forsake scholarship in favor of a frontal attack on the surface problems of the community, they risk losing the intellectual strength and creativity needed to untie the deeply complex knots of community need. The authors suggest that the rising challenge to universities, indeed the future course of universities, lies in resolving this dilemma, not by choosing one over the other but by finding how to couple the two in a philosophy of university action,[30] as we bravely march into the new millennium. And, of course, these concerns and actions must be pursued in terms of global dimensions. A fundamental advance in the roles of universities is to be found in their capacities for sharing both the burdens and understandings of these issues on a global basis.

ACKNOWLEDGMENTS

The authors wish to thank Naomi L. Ruff, PhD, ELS, for reviewing the manuscript and for her helpful suggestions and assistance with copyediting. The authors gratefully acknowledge the contribution of Ruth Bell, PhD, and Professor Sir Michael Marmot for the section, "How Can Universities Address the Social Determinants of Health?"

REFERENCES

1. Velji AM. International health. Beyond the year 2000. Infect Dis Clin North Am 1991;5(2):417–28.
2. Boyer EL. Scholarship reconsidered: priorities of the professoriate. Princeton (NJ): The Carnegie Foundation for the Advancement of Teaching; 1990.
3. White KL. Healing the schism: epidemiology, medicine, and the public's health. New York: Springer-Verlag; 1991.
4. Bryant JH. Educating tomorrow's doctors. World Health Forum 1993;14(3): 217–30 [discussion: 231–52].
5. Bryant JH, Marsh DR, Khan KS, et al. A developing country's university oriented toward strengthening health systems: challenges and results. Am J Public Health 1993;83(11):1537–43.
6. Palsdottir B, Neusy A. Global health: networking innovative academic institutions. Infect Dis Clin North Am 2011;25(2), in press.
7. Flexner A. Medical education in the United States and Canada. From the Carnegie Foundation for the Advancement of Teaching, Bulletin Number Four, 1910. Bull World Health Organ 2002;80(7):594–602.
8. Boelen C. A new paradigm for medical schools a century after Flexner's report. Bull World Health Organ 2002;80(7):592–3.
9. Showstack J, Fein O, Ford D, et al. Health of the public. The academic response. Health of the Public Mission Statement Working Group. JAMA 1992;267(18): 2497–502.
10. World Health Organization. The world health report 2000: health systems: improving performance. Geneva (Switzerland): World Health Organization; 2000.
11. Ijsselmuiden CB, Nchinda TC, Duale S, et al. Mapping Africa's advanced public health education capacity: the AfriHealth project. Bull World Health Organ 2007; 85(12):914–22.
12. Kalua F, Awotedu A, Kamwanja L, et al, editors. Science, technology and innovation for public health in Africa (monograph). Pretoria (Republic of South Africa): NEPAD Office of Science and Technology; 2009.
13. Velji AM. Preface: global health, global health education, and infectious disease. Infect Dis Clin North Am 2011;25(2):xiii–xxi.
14. World Health Organization. The role of universities in the strategies for health for all. Floor contributions, first plenary session: Dr. Sylla (Senegal). 37th World Health Assembly, technical discussions. 1984. Geneva (Switzerland). Available at: http://whqlibdoc.who.int/hq/1984/12738_(part1).pdf. Accessed August 6, 2010.
15. Lorntz B, Boissevain JR, Dillingham R, et al. A trans-university center for global health. Acad Med 2008;83(2):165–72.
16. Quinn TC. The Johns Hopkins Center for Global Health: transcending borders for world health. Acad Med 2008;83(2):134–42.
17. Koplan JP, Baggett RL. The Emory Global Health Institute: developing partnerships to improve health through research, training, and service. Acad Med 2008;83(2):128–33.
18. Velji AM. Global health education consortium: 20 years of leadership in global health and global health education. Infect Dis Clin North Am 2011;25(2), in press.
19. Vermund SH, Sahasrabuddhe VV, Khedkar S, et al. Building global health through a center-without-walls: the Vanderbilt Institute for Global Health. Acad Med 2008; 83(2):154–64.

20. Babich LP, Bicknell WJ, Culpepper L, et al. Social responsibility, international development, and institutional commitment: lessons from the Boston University experience. Acad Med 2008;83(2):143–7.
21. Olds GR. Geographic medicine: a new movement within international health. Acad Med 1989;64(4):190–2.
22. Williams RS, Casey PJ, Kamei RK, et al. A global partnership in medical education between Duke University and the National University of Singapore. Acad Med 2008;83(2):122–7.
23. Coates T, Debas H. The University of California Health Institute: a paradigm shift. Infect Dis Clin North Am 2011;25(3), in press.
24. Commission of the European Communities. Delivering on the modernisation agenda for universities: education, research and innovation. Brussels, May 5, 2006. Available at: http://ec.europa.eu/education/policies/2010/doc/comuniv2006_en.pdf. Accessed May 8, 2010.
25. Lambert R, Butler N. The future of European universities: renaissance or decay? London: Center for European Reform; 2006. Available at: www.cer.org.uk/pdf/p_67x_universities_decay_3.pdf. Accessed May 8, 2010.
26. Higher Education Funding Council for England. The higher education workforce framework 2010 Main report. 2010. Available at: http://www.hefce.ac.uk/pubs/hefce/2010/10_05a/10_05a.pdf. Accessed May 8, 2010.
27. Commission on Social Determinants of Health. Closing the gap in a generation: health equity through action on the social determinants of health: commission on social determinants of health final report. Geneva (Switzerland): World Health Organization; 2008. Available at: http://www.who.int/social_determinants/thecommission/finalreport/en/. Accessed May 8, 2010.
28. Marmot M, Friel S, Bell R, et al. Closing the gap in a generation: health equity through action on the social determinants of health. Lancet 2008;372(9650):1661–9.
29. Bryant JH. The role of Third World universities in health development. Asia Pac J Public Health 1991;5(2):123–30.
30. Bryant J. Health and the developing world. London: Cornell University Press; 1969.

Global Health Education Consortium: 20 Years of Leadership in Global Health and Global Health Education

Anvar Velji, MD, FRCP(c), FIDSA[a,b,*]

KEYWORDS

• Global health • Global health education • Consortium
• Networks • Competencies • Curriculum

“GHEC has played a critical role in the evolution of the global health movement. Its accomplishments over 20 years are evident in the growth of interest in the field.” (H. Debas, Chairman of the Board, Consortium of Universities for Global Health [CUGH], San Francisco, California, personal communication, Aug 1, 2010).

Founded in 1991, the Global Health Education Consortium (GHEC) is a network of universities and institutions committed to improving the health and human rights of underserved populations worldwide through improved education and training of the global workforce. Today, GHEC is recognized as the premier consortium of universities and is given credit for growth in the evolving global health movement in general and in education and advocacy in particular.

GHEC started out with meetings and planning strategies and retreats among faculties and administrators from several universities keenly mindful of the rapidly changing global health landscape and the need for basic change in global health education.[1,2]

GHEC was originally limited to medical schools in its North American base, but in 2005 it extended its membership to other health professions and expanded its

This work was supported by funding from Kaiser Permanente.
[a] Department of Infectious Disease, Kaiser Permanente, South Sacramento, 6600 Bruceville Road, Sacramento, CA 95823, USA
[b] Department of Infectious Disease, School of Medicine, University of California, Davis, CA, USA
* Department of Infectious Disease, Kaiser Permanente, South Sacramento, 6600 Bruceville Road, Sacramento, CA 95823.
E-mail address: Anvarali.Velji@kp.org

Infect Dis Clin N Am 25 (2011) 323–335
doi:10.1016/j.idc.2011.02.003 id.theclinics.com

programs globally. Today its institutional members include more than 100 universities, as well as nongovernmental organizations (NGO) and individual members in North America, Central America and the Caribbean, Africa, and Asia.

In the 1990s, in anticipation of the new millennium, efforts increased to popularize global health and global health education strongly linked to a deep sense of commitment, morality, fairness, and social justice. The epiphany and concept for launching a university consortium took place in 1990 in Washington, DC; the initial focus was on medical schools, and the consortium was dedicated to furthering global health development and education as a means for training the workforce with idealism and for fulfilling the needs of the marginalized both at home and abroad.[1] The inaugural meeting was hosted by the University of Arizona in 1991 and officially launched the International Health Medical Education Consortium. The organization subsequently changed its name and is now known as GHEC. In the subsequent discussion, GHEC is used as the preferred name of the organization, although the name change did not occur until 2004. Faculty, program administrators from 24 US universities, global health program directors, and individuals committed to raising the profile of training in global health were in attendance. The nascent state of global health within medical schools was evident in the title of the keynote address at the inaugural meeting: "Why International Health [global health] in the US Schools of Medicine?"[2]

This current article was prompted by several recent developments, as well as a desire to catalog some dramatic changes in global health and global health education in the new millennium and to document some of the major contributions of the consortium and its pervasive influence. Before the founding of GHEC, most universities in North America had long been involved in global health, albeit sporadically, through their students, faculty, and other educators, at the individual, divisional, departmental, or institution level. The involvement was mostly focused on developing curricula, research in tropical diseases, or setting up epidemiology units. A major exception was the Network of Community Oriented Health Science Centers,[3] now known as The Network for Unity of Health (TUFH), and the efforts of Canadian universities through their health science departments. TUFH was founded in Jamaica in 1977 by the World Health Organization (WHO) to help educational institutions provide future health workers with training that was relevant to the health needs of a given population. At that point in time, only 1.5% of medical schools had adopted innovative programs and teaching methods.[4] Among the developed nations, the United States was conspicuous in its meager contribution to international medical education, especially when compared with the socialist-bloc nations. However, the American Medical Association (AMA) and its members had been active in international health from the time of the Second World War. The AMA also supported the work of the WHO and the International Refugee Organization, and in the United States it had been a major force in establishing the National Council for International Health (NCIH), now the Global Health Council.[5] By the early 1990s, interest in international health was increasing once again among medical students and faculty at many universities.

From 1969 to 1981 there was an increase of 63% in US health professionals working overseas, and church-related organizations, corporations, and universities were increasingly becoming more active.[6] US corporate involvement increased to develop the health workforce in the oil-rich nations, and Baker and colleagues[6] estimated that the future demand for high-level international health workers would be only in the range of 1500. As a result, Baker and colleagues[6] felt that the involvement of the United States in international health did not constitute "a drain on the US physician supply." [6] In an international health survey performed by the Educational Committee on Foreign Medical Graduates (ECFMG), nearly every US medical school reported having international programs, which ranged from aerospace medicine, biometrics, and curriculum design to urology and virology.[7]

In 1974, Case Western Reserve University established the first division of geographic medicine within the department of medicine at the University Hospital in Cleveland, Ohio. This movement was new within international health. Historically, the study of tropical diseases had been located outside the mainstream of medical science and relegated to schools of public health.[8]

GHEC was founded in the context of this global education scene. However, there were other major changes on the global scene that had eluded many educators. The author subsequently reviews some of these changes.

In 1989, there was a vibrant movement, which I called the Global Health Care Revolution, with awakening of ideas, ideals, and actions in global health and global health education; still, not all the players in the health systems and schools of medicine were involved.[1,5] One major function of the newly formed consortium was to help expand the horizons of medical schools, which were functioning primarily as educators and researchers isolated from social realities. It was hoped that the schools would eventually become active collaborators with WHO and provide moral, spiritual, and social leadership in bringing health to the global human being, a term I preferred over the global citizen, abroad and at home.[1] I thought that the movement was historically significant, that it would bring together under one organization all of the diverse international activities of all American medical schools, and that the organization would have leverage at national and international levels in policymaking and in devising curricula. It was hoped that it would also address the long-standing curricular needs with regard to clinical sites, funding issues, curricular changes, academic credits, career tracks, and resource sharing for predoctoral, doctoral, and postdoctoral students in international health (now known as global health) by providing a clearing house.[1]

I thought that the concept and content of international health needed to be expanded. The ongoing HIV epidemic had made it clear that the welfare and health interests of various nations were interlocked, and curricular changes at graduate and postgraduate levels were critically needed to address these global issues in which we were suddenly immersed unprepared. In addition, economics, communications, and various sciences had already emerged as strong global forces that would impact health going forward. Those who were practitioners in the field of international health (global health) needed to shape the new world and become part of the vision.[5] This action would require a reappraisal of then-existing concepts of international health simply as dealings between nations to provide health aid and technological assistance to developing economies. The next task was to define this new concept of global health. For me it meant health care that was targeted to the global human being, shared between nations and encompassing multiple disciplines and sciences. Global health included primary health care, public health, nutrition, maternal-child and women's health, geographic and tropical medicine, infectious disease, and so on. It had to have a *moral* and *spiritual* component, in keeping with the concept of health for all.[5] Moreover, as our globe shrinks, I thought that collaboration was required among universities of the North, South, East, and West in all combinations and also required training international health human resources as well as formation of a university consortium for global health.[5]

DEFINING GLOBAL HEALTH AND ITS CONTOURS

As a first step in defining the new philosophy and the emerging discipline of global health, my works already used creative new terminology in 1991 and 1992, such as the "global human being," "global person," "global health professional," "Global Health Care Revolution," "good global health," and "global health problems." These were the transitional years when the terminology of international health and global health overlapped. As the next step, 49 experts in global health and global health education were invited specifically to summarize then-current challenges, problems with logistics, and concerns in global health, global health education, and more specifically to share their ideals, ideas, actions, and vision for global health beyond the year 2000. These experts brought in experience from their various roles as educators; ethicists; heads of global health programs; environmentalists; scientists; and researchers in fields, including infectious disease, tropical medicine, public health, anthropology, ethics, travel medicine, primary health care, population, the environment, women's health, toxicology, aging, population displacement, informatics, and many more. NGOs, foundations, and a wide variety of programs and institutions were represented, including the US Centers of Disease Control and Prevention, the World Bank, WHO, United Nations Development Program, National Institutes of Health, United States Agency for International Development, International Clinical Epidemiology Network, NCIH, and the newly formed GHEC. Thus, for the first time, to our knowledge, the contours, contents, and philosophy of global health had been outlined. These outlines supplemented or formed the basis of several of the global health curricula of GHEC schools in North America and thus became the first textbooks on global health,[9,10] exploring a different approach than the extant textbook on international health by Paul Basch.[11]

In the quest for involving universities in global health in a formal way, articles were invited that covered how to set up academic programs in international health.[12,13] Here the authors outlined the rationale for establishing a formal, institution-wide program in global health and offered broad guidelines for an institute or center for global health. They further articulated the need for institutional policy, formulations of an organizational framework and assessment of institutional capacity, and objectives relevant to health development agendas. Several universities who were already members of GHEC, such as the University of Indiana, Tulane, University of Arizona, and Case Western Reserve, focused on their unique global health programs.[14–17] A robust program also existed at Yale University in the department of internal medicine.[18]

GHEC AND THE ROLE OF UNIVERSITIES IN GLOBAL HEALTH AND GLOBAL HEALTH EDUCATION

Health agendas struggled for a place on the development agendas in most countries in the 1990s (even after Alma Ata, a similar fate befell global health in academic centers in North America). GHEC priority areas were outlined during the GHEC Governing Council retreat in 1993; however, Jack Bryant, MD, both a GHEC consultant and member, proposed an expanded perspective of GHEC that included roles of universities, health development, health policy, health systems development, and patterns of disease, among others. He also noted, "individual interests were giving way to common purpose within the new organization."[19] In his keynote address at the 1994 GHEC Annual Meeting held at the University of Texas-El Paso, Bryant further elucidated the role of GHEC in transforming universities and involving them in development. Things have changed since then because of several robust commitments by networks, such as GHEC, whose students, faculty, and administrators performed rigorous advocacy at all levels, resulting in proliferation of Global Health Centers of Excellence and innovative schools committed to several key principles of health for all.

The success of an organization is measured by the strength of its volunteerism and the outcomes of its mission, vision, goals, influence in the field or fields it chooses to influence, and ability to change despite the most severe challenges and constraints. In the case of GHEC, the efforts have largely rested on the backbone of faculty, students, residents, and administrator volunteers at allopathic and osteopathic medical schools, schools of public health, and nursing schools. Several prominent successes and ongoing efforts over the last 2 decades include promotion and facilitation of the following:

1. Global health and global health education based on the principles and philosophy of health for all in universities, schools of public health, nursing, and allied sciences in a multidimensional manner crossing borders and disciplines (GHEC programs have stressed that there is no difference in how health and health care is perceived and delivered between our populations here and those abroad. Equity, fairness, and human rights have been the pillars of this endeavor.)
2. Leadership and training of the global health workforce through education here and abroad
3. Networking between individuals, students, faculty, and their institutions and collaborators both in the Americas and abroad on the basis of mutual respect, trust, and professionalism and with a focus on their combined, agreed-upon goals.

The earliest committees of GHEC, founded in 1992, consisted of curriculum development, linkages and networking, student placement, clinical sites, cross-cultural student residency task force, and membership.[20] By the midyear annual GHEC meeting in Arlington, Virginia, 51 universities were present in addition to the American Medical Student Association (AMSA), US Department of State, Harvard and Johns Hopkins Schools of Public Health, Indian Health Service, NCIH (now the Global Health Council), and Pan American Health Organization (PAHO). GHEC held several of its annual meetings to run concurrently with those of the American Association of Medical Colleges (AAMC). At the 1993 annual AAMC meeting, GHEC presented a panel on "Cross-Cultural Training in US Medical Schools–Lessons learned from International Health." GHEC and AAMC representatives met to develop educational objectives for culturally competent care and global health training with the goal of possibly incorporating these objectives into AAMC accreditation criteria.

Over the years, GHEC members have participated in and made many contributions to other organizations concerned with global health issues. Relationships with such organizations as the Institute of Medicine (IOM), PAHO, WHO, TUFH, AAMC, American Public Health Association (APHA), American Society of Tropical Medicine and Hygiene, ECFMG, Global Health Council, and the World Bank provide opportunities for sharing expertise and for collaboration or coordination of projects of mutual interest. Jack Bryant, MD, subsequently the chair of the International Health Section of the APHA (1995–1996), initiated an effort to incorporate his global thinking into the APHA strategic planning process. Bryant also attempted to reestablish cooperative relationships with NCIH, IOM, National Academy of Science, and other entities.[21] Both the Infectious Disease Society and the American Society of Tropical Medicine also now have sections of global health largely because of the advocacy of GHEC members and others involved in global health.

GLOBAL HEALTH EDUCATION CONSORTIUM AND SOCIAL ACCOUNTABILITY OF UNIVERSITIES AND SCHOOLS OF MEDICINE

GHEC has been a major supporter of the concepts and philosophies of equity, responsiveness, responsibility, and social accountability of universities in general and medical schools in particular. It emphasizes at its annual conferences and in publications how to train socially accountable professionals who will be *change agents* in their societies to improve equitable distribution of health care resources and who will be leaders in advocating for better health care for all and in building stronger health care systems. A GHEC past president coauthored a seminal work on social accountability.[22] The Training for Health Equity Network (THEnet), a sister organization of GHEC, played a major role at the recent Consensus Conference on Social Accountability in Medical Schools in South Africa, along with leading global educational leadership and organizations, such as the WHO, Foundation for Advancement of International Medical Education and Research (FAIMER), and the World Federation of Medical Schools.

GHEC UNIVERSITIES AND NGO NETWORKS

The author offers several examples to illustrate how some of the earliest GHEC academic health centers have networked to improve global health in its several dimensions.

Shoulder to Shoulder (Hombro a Hombro)

Departments of family and community medicine within academic centers in the United States have been leaders in global health education[23] and have played a significant role in the development of GHEC and its mission. The University of Cincinnati Family Medicine residency program began to officially offer global health training in 1991. Since then, their successful model, Shoulder to Shoulder, has now been replicated in 6 geographic regions.

The Moi-Indiana University Partnership in Health

The Moi University Faculty of Health Sciences and the Indiana University School of Medicine have formed a model of a successful partnership over several decades. This partnership is focused on development of leaders in sub-Saharan Africa and in the United States.[14] Like the University of North Carolina before it, Indiana University hosted the GHEC Secretariat for many years.

Global Health Fellowships

In 1995, 3 GHEC Schools—the Universities of Wisconsin, Colorado, and Rochester—and the AMSA Foundation joined to develop a global health fellowship for US medical students and to develop a core curriculum in global health. Sixty students participated and completed their field experiences at several universities in middle-income and low-income countries. The partner universities and institutions were Universidad Nacional Autonoma de Honduras; Universidad de Valle, Columbia; Chiang Mai University, Thailand; University of the Witwatersrand, South Africa; Moi University, Kenya; Christian Medical College, India; and King Edward Medical College, Pakistan. These schools were selected based on the strengths of their community-oriented primary care, the faculty's willingness to supervise students, safety, and logistical factors.[24]

Recently, Afia Bora (Good Health), a more robust fellowship program to train global health leaders has been created among 8 participating institutions, 4 in Africa and 4 in the United States, to help build the workforce and leadership capacity in Africa.[25]

Child Family Health International

In late 2007, GHEC partnered with Child Family Health International (CFHI; http://cfhi.org/), a San Francisco-based NGO. CFHI was founded by Evaleen Jones, MD, who was then a resident and also served on the GHEC board. CFHI currently operates more than 20 programs in 5 countries.

Training for Health Equity Network (THEnet)

In 2007, GHEC received funding from the Atlantic Philanthropies to assess how selected schools of health sciences and medicine that had been established specifically to address the health needs of the underserved were meeting this obligation. These schools are located in different regions of the world but have a social mandate and strong community engagement in common. They have embraced social accountability principles at the core of their mission while adopting somewhat different strategies to respond to the divergent contexts in which they operate. The schools include the Northern Ontario School of Medicine in Canada; the School of Health Sciences and Medicine at Walter Sisulu University in South Africa; the Latin American School of Medicine in Cuba; the Comprehensive Community Physician Training Program in Venezuela; Ateneo de Zamboanga University School of Medicine and the School of Health Sciences in Leyte in the Philippines; and Flinders University School of Health Sciences and Medicine and the James Cook Faculty of Medicine, Health and Molecular Sciences in Australia. In 2008, the leadership of these schools met in La Havana, Cuba, to provide an opportunity for each of these schools to break their isolation and be linked with like-minded institutions. They also recognized the need to collaborate, pool and share resources, develop new evaluation standards, and create a solid evidence base to underpin and disseminate their work. The schools decided to create a new independent organization, which was incorporated in 2009. THEnet is a global network of socially accountable schools of health sciences and medicine sharing a core commitment to achieving equity in health care and health outcomes through quality health education, service, and action-oriented research that is responsive to the needs of, and embedded in, undeserved communities and health care systems. By acting as a resource and open platform for outcome-oriented health professional schools in under-resourced areas, THEnet seeks to optimize the contribution of health profession schools to improving health outcomes in the communities they serve.[26]

GLOBAL HEALTH CENTERS OF EXPERTISE AND EXCELLENCE

There has been an explosion of Centers of Expertise and Excellence in Global Health at several North American universities to coordinate the multidisciplinary activities and interests from transuniversity to intrauniversity research, teaching, service, advocacy, policy development, and global health diplomacy.[27,28]

GLOBAL HEALTH EDUCATION CONSORTIUM AND THE ROLE OF STUDENTS

Over the last two decades there have been close ties between GHEC and individual students and student organizations. An invited personal communication from the chair of the International Health Section, Linda Barthauer, February, 1991 of AMSA was presented at the inaugural meeting by the author (AV), indicating the strong interest of the AMSA and the International Federation of Medical Students Associations (IFMSA) and leadership to be involved with the new consortium. Following this meeting a student-resident liaison committee (Student and Resident Advocacy Committee) was formed, and by the following annual meeting the consortium invited one student and one resident to be part of the governing council.[29]

GHEC continues its strong commitment to students as evidenced by its student advisory committee, currently with representation from 6 student organizations and student representation on its board of directors. The linkages bring the energy, ideas, and perspectives of future global health leaders and policy makers to the consortium's policies and programs.

MAJOR RECENT GHEC INITIATIVES

A Survey of US Medical School Participation in Global Health Activities

Several critical surveys have been performed by GHEC schools, such as assessing medical schools' preparation of students for overseas practice.[30] In 2007, the Trans-University Alliance of Institutes Networking for Global Health (TrainGH) developed a framework and development survey to assess the need for a transuniversity alliance to address capacity building of global health professionals in low-resource areas around the world. GHEC, The Fogarty International Center, and the University of Virginia prepared and performed the survey. As part of the TrainGH Project, GHEC and the Center for Global Health of the University of Virginia also performed a Internet-based search in late 2007 and early 2008 for university-based and college-based global health programs in North America. This search identified 192 programs. A bibliography with 47 recent relevant citations was also compiled for capacity building of global health professionals in developing countries through inter-university partnerships.[31] A survey on international programs performed recently by FAIMER, GHEC, and AMSA indicated that a variety of international opportunities are available to students at US medical schools.[32]

Annual and Regional Conferences

GHEC has an annual conference in rotating venues. From 1993 to 2009 the conference was held in the Caribbean, Central America, Canada, and the United States. The 2010 conference was hosted by the Instituto Nacional de Salud Pública (INSP) in Mexico. Conference features include plenary and breakout presentations, student posters, NGO exhibits, and awards for distinguished service and student accomplishments. The annual conference provides an invaluable means for updating information, sharing ideas, recognizing accomplishments, and networking. The reach of the annual conference is greatly extended by 3 to 5 regional conferences held each year and hosted by GHEC member institutions in collaboration with GHEC.

The 19th GHEC conference and the first Annual Latin American and Caribbean Global Health Conference were hosted in Mexico by INSP. An agreement was reached between representatives from 7 nations present at the meeting (Brazil, Argentina, Chile, Mexico, Cuba, Peru, and Nicaragua) to create a networking alliance (The Latin American Global Health Alliance [Alianza Latino Americana de Salud Global (ALASAG)]) to address global health needs by fostering collaborative alliances among experts from the region's academic institutions through an articulated program of human resource development, research, and technical cooperation. ALASAG will enable a coordinated regional effort to address global health challenges and to strengthen human resources and research, knowledge, and skills required for the management of the global health.[33–35] In 2011, GHEC, CUGH, and the Canadian Society of International Health will be holding a joint conference in Montreal. Many of the recent conferences have been cosponsored by major organizations, including the Fogarty International Center; International Development Research Center (Canada); PAHO; The Lancet; Kaiser Family Foundation; the Bill and Melinda Gates Foundation; several partner universities, including the University of California San Francisco, University of California Davis, University of Washington Seattle, University of Toronto, and Harvard; Kaiser Permanente; the Margaret Kendrick Blodgett Foundation; and several pharmaceutical industry foundations.

Global Health Curriculum and Competencies

From its founding, GHEC has focused on 4 components of global health education: curriculum, instruction, experience in the field, and evaluation (competency and certification). GHEC universities and institutions have long held that the curriculum should be mission and service driven and mindful of societal needs and goals. The crucible for developing, testing, and improving such curricula is the real world of poverty, societal discrimination, human rights violations, limited resources, chronic conditions, emerging and reemerging infections, environmental degradation, and other societal challenges. The field of action is the inner cities, native reservations, migrant health centers, refugee camps, and other underserved and neglected areas both here and abroad. The curriculum is thus more than a plan that determines an educational experience, parceled into discrete learning objectives in several domains and achievement of certain competencies aimed at satisfying examining bodies for professional certification. Developing curriculum objectives within the Accreditation Council for Graduate Medical Education competency-based framework ensures that global health curricula encompass all domains important to resident education, not only medical knowledge and patient care but also domains of professionalism, communication, and practice-based learning, which are all highly relevant to global health. Competency-based curriculum objectives can guide both the program and the individual resident toward achieving well-defined, appropriate, and realistic educational goals during residency. Finally, these curriculum objectives allow for effective evaluation of resident performance, including faculty and mentor assessment and resident self-assessment. Recently, core competencies in global health have been defined by a joint committee of experts from the Association of Faculties of Medicine of Canada Resource Group on Global Health and GHEC.[36] GHEC members have also been active in developing the curriculum recommendations for the Family Medicine Residency Programs.[37]

Global Health Modules

More than 80 draft eLearning modules are currently available for use online, and about 60 more are in preparation.[38] All modules will be peer and student reviewed before the final versions are posted on the GHEC Web site. Future plans call for continuing education and certification.

Global Health Bibliography

The Global Health Bibliography, initiated in 2002 and revised, updated, and greatly expanded by a team of students, residents, and faculty in 2007 to 2008, focuses on global health classics and current articles in 27 topic categories, with approximately 820 citations.[39] It will be expanded to include a wider variety of teaching resources.

Global Health Student and Resident Guidebook

The first edition of this guidebook, published in 2008, entailed a collaborative effort with input from residency directors. The guide includes a rationale for pursuing global health, opportunities and challenges in global health, selection of residency programs, surveys, and draft competency standards for pediatric residency.[40] A new and expanded edition was just published in 2011.

The Global Health Curriculum Guidebook

The global health curriculum has been a long-standing concern and interest of GHEC schools. In 2006, GHEC collaborated with 3 student organizations (AMSA, International Federation of Medical Students' Associations [IFMSA-USA], and the Canadian

Federation of Medical Students) and CFHI to prepare a guidebook designed to help universities to develop or improve a global health curriculum. Now in its second edition, this guidebook was revised in 2008.[41]

Global Health Directors Network

A Global Health Directors Network was launched in 2008 at the GHEC annual conference in Sacramento, California. With more than 60 members, the network seeks to facilitate program director exchange on common problems and to promote best practices in the development and management of global health educational programs.

Global Health Textbooks

GHEC authors and editors continue to set the trend for excellence, as evidenced by multiple recent resources.[42,43] Recently, GHEC launched a global health textbook evaluation project in which 37 faculty and student reviewers assessed the quality and readability of 5 introductory global health textbooks according to 5 evaluation criteria. The findings will be published and help prospective purchasers make their choices among a variety of textbook options.

GHEC Awards

GHEC established the Distinguished Service Award in 1993, followed by the Christopher Krogh Award, and in 2008, The Lancet-GHEC Award for students to recognize outstanding research and community service projects. In addition, 3 Velji Awards recognize global health excellence: Teaching Excellence in Global Health, Emerging Leader in Global Health, and the Project of the Year.[44]

SUMMARY

GHEC continues to be the leader in the twenty-first century in addressing and advocating for education reform for health professionals with more training and opportunities, curriculum development, and competency certification throughout the world based on principles of equity, quality, and access.[45,46] The recent formation of the CUGH is fortuitous and timely. CUGH complements GHEC in the areas of education policy development, political level advocacy, research, and extension of global health within universities. The transdisciplinary and interdisciplinary involvement of universities are critical in solving global health challenges through the power of universities and schools of public health, nursing, and other allied fields.[47]

ACKNOWLEDGMENTS

The author wishes to recognize Thomas Hall, MD for many years of service to GHEC in various capacities, including executive directorship (pro bono) as well as nurturing several GHEC product initiatives, and Andre Jacques Neusy, MD for his leadership at GHEC during a critical period in its transition and for contributing the section on THEnet in this article. This article is dedicated to all of our students and faculty who made the GHEC dream a reality. The author also wishes to thank Dr Thomas Hall for reviewing the manuscript and for his helpful suggestions and Naomi L. Ruff, PhD, ELS for copy-editing assistance.

REFERENCES

1. Velji A. International health. West J Med 1991;155(3):308–9.

2. Velji AM. Keynote address: why international health in US medical schools–and how do we communicate the vision to our constituents. Paper presented at: Inaugural meeting on International Health in Colleges of Medicine. Tucson (AZ), February 28–March 2, 1991.
3. Stuck C, Bickley LS, Wallace N, et al. International health medical education consortium. Its history, philosophy, and role in medical education and health development. Infect Dis Clin North Am 1995;9(2):419–23.
4. Schmidt HG, Neufeld VR, Nooman ZM, et al. Network of community-oriented educational institutions for the health sciences. Acad Med 1991;66(5):259–63.
5. Velji AM. International health. Beyond the year 2000. Infect Dis Clin North Am 1991;5(2):417–28.
6. Baker TD, Weisman C, Piwoz E. US physicians in international health. Report of a current survey. JAMA 1984;251(4):502–4.
7. Asper S, Steel W, editors. Directory of international programs and projects of US schools of medicine, dentistry, pharmacy, and public health. Philadelphia: Educational Commission for Foreign Medical Graduates; 1988.
8. Olds GR. Geographic medicine: a new movement within international health. Acad Med 1989;64(4):190–2.
9. Velji AM, editor. International health. Beyond the year 2000, vol. 5. Philadelphia: WB Saunders Co; 1991. Infect Dis Clin North Am, No. 2.
10. Velji AM, editor. International health, beyond the year 2000, vol. 9. Philadelphia: W. B. Saunders; 1995. Infect Dis Clin North Am, No. 2.
11. Basch PF. Textbook of international health. New York: Oxford University Press; 1990.
12. Bryant JH, Zuberi RW, Thaver IH. Alma Ata and health for all by the year 2000. The roles of academic institutions. Infect Dis Clin North Am 1991;5(2): 403–16.
13. Sajid AW, Wunderlich M. How to set up your program in international health. Infect Dis Clin North Am 1991;5(2):393–402.
14. Einterz RM, Kelley CR, Mamlin JJ, et al. Partnerships in international health. The Indiana University-Moi University experience. Infect Dis Clin North Am 1995;9(2):453–5.
15. Chiller TM, De Mieri P, Cohen I. International health training. The Tulane experience. Infect Dis Clin North Am 1995;9(2):439–43.
16. Torjesen H. An international health story from Case Western Reserve University. Infect Dis Clin North Am 1995;9(2):433–7.
17. Pust RE, Moher SP. Medical education for international health. The Arizona experience. Infect Dis Clin North Am 1995;9(2):445–51.
18. Gupta AR, Wells CK, Horwitz RI, et al. The International Health Program: the fifteen-year experience with Yale University's Internal Medicine Residency Program. Am J Trop Med Hyg 1999;61(6):1019–23.
19. IHMEC. Minutes. IHMEC Governing Council Retreat, University of Wisconsin, Madison, April 16, 1993.
20. IHMEC. Minutes. IHMEC Auxiliary Meeting. Washington, DC, June 15, 1992.
21. Growth of International Health: an analysis and history. Washington, DC: American Public Health Association; 2003. Available at: http://www.apha.org/NR/rdonlyres/9F224874-D174-4DBC-9418-EEDE49BC0D08/0/InternationalHealthBook.pdf. Accessed March 27, 2011.
22. Boelen C, Heck J. Defining and measuring the social accountability of medical schools, HRH 95.7. Geneva (Switzerland): World Health Organization; 1995. Available on request from Division of Organization and Management of Health Systems.

23. Heck JE, Bazemore A, Diller P. The shoulder to shoulder model-channeling medical volunteerism toward sustainable health change. Fam Med 2007;39(9): 644–50.
24. Haq C, Rothenberg D, Gjerde C, et al. New world views: preparing physicians in training for global health work. Fam Med 2000;32(8):566–72.
25. Farquhar C, Nathanson N. The Afya Bora Consortium: an Africa-US partnership to train leaders in global health. Infect Dis Clin North Am 2011;25(2), in press.
26. Pálsdóttir B, Neusy A. Global health: networking innovative academic institutions. Infect Dis Clin North Am 2011;25(2), in press.
27. Kanter SL. Global health initiative. Acad Med 2008;83(2, theme issue):115–98.
28. Bryant JH, Velji AM. Global health and the role of universities in the twenty-first century. Infect Dis Clin North Am 2011;25(2), in press.
29. IHMEC. Governing Council Meeting Minutes. IHMEC Auxiliary Meeting. Washington, DC, June 14, 1992.
30. Heck JE, Wedemeyer D. A survey of American medical schools to assess their preparation of students for overseas practice. Acad Med 1991;66(2):78–81.
31. Global Health Education Consortium. Trans-University Alliance of Institutes Networking for Global Health (TrainGH). Available at: http://globalhealtheducation.org/aboutus/Pages/ProjectsServices.aspx#8. Accessed November 22, 2010.
32. McKinley DW, Williams SR, Norcini JJ, et al. International exchange programs and U.S. medical schools. Acad Med 2008;83(10 Suppl):S53–7.
33. Alliances for Global Health Education: learning from South-South Collaboration. 2010 GHEC Conference. 2010. Cuernavaca (Mexico). Available at: http://globalhealth.kff.org/Multimedia/2010/April/10/GHEC-Keynote.aspx. Accessed February 2, 2011.
34. Reunión de establecimiento de ALASAG [Meeting for the establishment of ALASAG]. Salud Global Boletin Informativo (Electronic bulletin), 2010;4:3 [in Spanish].
35. Salgado de Snyder VN, DeMaria LM. Latin American Global Health Alliance: building collaborations across the region [poster 02.61]. CUGH Meeting, 2010. University of Washington, Seattle, April 3–5, 2009. Available at: http://www.cugh.org/sites/default/files/2010-annual/program-book.pdf. Accessed March 27, 2011.
36. Arthur MAM, Battat R, Brewer TF. Teaching the basics: core competencies in global health. Infect Dis Clin North Am 2011;25(2), in press.
37. American Academy of Family Physicians. Recommended Curriculum Guidelines for Family Medicine Residents Global Health [AAFP Reprint No. 287] 2010. Available at: http://www.aafp.org/online/etc/medialib/aafp_org/documents/about/rap/curriculum/globalhealth.Par.0001.File.tmp/Reprint287.pdf. Accessed September 29, 2010.
38. Global Health Education Consortium. Teaching modules. Available at: http://globalhealtheducation.org/Modules/SitePages/Home.aspx. Accessed February 9, 2011.
39. Global Health Education Consortium. Global health bibliography. Available at: http://globalhealtheducation.org/resources/Pages/GlobalHealthBibliography.aspx. Accessed February 9, 2011.
40. Evert J, Mautner D, Hoffman J. Developing global health curricula: a guidebook for US medical schools. Available at: http://globalhealthedu.org/PublicDocs/Developing GH Curricula_Guidebook for US Medical Schools.pdf. Accessed March 27, 2011.
41. Evert J, Stewart C, Chan K, et al. Developing residency training in global health: a guidebook. San Francisco (CA): Global Health Education Consortium; 2008. Available at: http://globalhealtheducation.org/PublicDocs/GHEC%20Residency%20Guidebook.pdf. Accessed March 27, 2011.

42. Drain PK. Caring for the world: a guidebook to global health opportunities. Toronto: University of Toronto Press; 2009.
43. Markle WH, Fisher MA, Smego RA. Understanding global health. New York: McGraw-Hill Medical; 2007.
44. Global Health Education Consortium. Awards. Available at: http://globalhealtheducation.org/resources/pages/awards.aspx. Accessed May 02, 2011.
45. Drain PK, Primack A, Hunt DD, et al. Global health in medical education: a call for more training and opportunities. Acad Med 2007;82(3):226–30.
46. Houpt ER, Pearson RD, Hall TL. Three domains of competency in global health education: recommendations for all medical students. Acad Med 2007;82(3): 222–5.
47. Merson MH, Chapman Page K. The dramatic expansion of university engagement in global health: implications for U.S. policy: a report by the CSIS Global Health Policy Center. Washington, DC: Center for Strategic and International Studies; 2009. Available at: http://www.csis.org/media/csis/pubs/090420_merson_dramaticexpansion.pdf. Accessed February 12, 2010.

Global Health: Networking Innovative Academic Institutions

Björg Pálsdóttir, MPA[a], André-Jacques Neusy, MD, DTM&H[b,c,*]

KEYWORDS

- Socially accountable schools • Health workforce
- Learning network • Outcome evaluation

The impact of globalization—the accelerated global integration of economic, political, cultural, social, and religious systems—on health is profound and complex. Health risks can be exported and imported like any commodity, and so can health workers. And poverty everywhere generates insidious public health risks for populations everywhere. Factors such as culture, trade, environment, demographics, access to care, gender roles, and human rights impact the health of all communities. The massive increase in the movement of goods, services, capital, ideas, innovations, individuals, and microbes does not only affect health. It also influences health system capacity, various aspects of service delivery, health labor markets, the health industry, the generation and flow of research and information.[1]

Global pandemics such as human immunodeficiency virus (HIV)/acquired immunodeficiency syndrome (AIDS) thrust global health to the forefront of overseas development assistance in the 1990s. Yet, despite quadrupling in global health funding,[2,3] health inequities within and among countries persist.[4] Initially, the bulk of global health funding went to biomedical research and interventions. However, the deficit and maldistribution of the health workforce rapidly emerged as a bottleneck in most regions. Health workforce density is an important variable in key health indicators such as maternal, infant, and under-5 mortality rates.[5,6] The World Health Organization (WHO) estimates that the global deficit of doctors, nurses, and

This work was supported by ACT grant 17391 from Atlantic Charitable Trust.
The authors have nothing to disclose.

[a] Program Development, Training for Health Equity Network, 54, Rue du Fosty, B-1470 Baisy-Thy, Belgium
[b] Global Health Education Consortium, USA
[c] Training for Health Equity Network, 54, Rue du Fosty, B-1470 Baisy-Thy, Belgium
* Corresponding author. Training for Health Equity Network, 54, Rue du Fosty, B-1470 Baisy-Thy, Belgium.
E-mail address: aj.neusy@gmail.com

Infect Dis Clin N Am 25 (2011) 337–346
doi:10.1016/j.idc.2011.02.001 id.theclinics.com
0891-5520/11/$ – see front matter

midwives to be around 2.4 million, and several countries will have to increase their workforce by about 140%to achieve adequate health coverage to increase life expectancy.[7] Beyond the shortage of health workers, another global challenge is the migration of health workers to urban and wealthier areas and across borders.[8] The brain drain takes its greatest toll on the most vulnerable populations, particularly those living in rural and poor urban communities.

While addressing maldistribution is a complex challenge and cannot be addressed only by health profession schools, they have a central role to play. They can implement strategies and programs that maximize the likelihood of appropriately trained professionals choosing to work in underserved areas. Predominant models of health workforce education are not producing the people, research, and services needed to expand universal health coverage.[4] Even in the United States, more than 65 million people live in areas with a shortage of primary care providers.[9] Yet trends in graduate US medical education suggest that 15% fewer primary care physicians will be entering the workforce, and more older providers are retiring at a time when the need is growing.[10] Unfortunately, gaps in medically underserved areas in high-income countries are often partially filled by medical graduates from poor countries with even greater needs. The estimates in loss of public investment in medical education in Africa due to out-migration are $500 million per year.[11] Migration of doctors also affects the ability of medical schools in Africa to retain their teaching faculties, further compounding the health workforce challenges.[12]

Maldistribution is only a part of the challenge in health profession education. The Independent Global Commission on Education of Health Professionals for the 21st Century, in a recent report calls for the redesign of institutional and educational strategies within the framework of health system reform. The suggested reforms are related to where, how, and what students are being taught.[4]

Many low-income countries are modeling their medical education programs on those in Europe or the United States. In 2003, the Institute of Medicine of the National Academies of Science called for more "outcome-based education system that better prepares clinicians to meet both the needs of patients and the requirements of a changing health system."[13] A new Carnegie Foundation study found that medical training in the United States lacks flexibility, longitudinal clinical exposure, and focus on patient populations, the health system. and efficiency. It claims that medical training is excessively centered on in-patient clinical experiences in tertiary care settings with inadequate capacity to support teaching.[14] The 2 reports underpin the lack of alignment between changing needs of health systems and societies and the strategies and programs of health profession institutions.

While most health education institutions have missions and goals related to improving health in their communities, few—in the north or the south—hold themselves accountable for producing outcomes aligned with health workforce, priority health, and health system needs. For example, education program design and evaluation objectives rarely focus on the practice and location of graduates, career development opportunities, or impact of research on policies and practice. Seldom do they attempt to evaluate factors that are difficult to measure such as the effect of institutional values on the career choices or practice of graduates.

It is not only schools that fall short of measuring their contribution to improving health. Today's accreditation standards do not adequately assess the impact of medical schools on the public good,[15] and there are scant comparable international data on relationships between current accreditation processes and outcomes.[16] The calls for more evidence on what works and for more social accountability of health professions institutions grow louder.[4,15,17–19]

THE TRAINING FOR HEALTH EQUITY NETWORK

Yet, below the radar screen several innovative institutions in rural, remote, and underserved regions of Africa, Asia, Australia, and the Americas are striving towards social accountability. They offer inspiring leadership and invaluable lessons of the potential for institutional impact, particularly in medically underserved populations. Perhaps not coincidentally, some of the most innovative efforts developed in areas with great needs and limited resources. Many emerged from or were influenced by the movement towards primary care and the Alma Ata Declaration of "Health for All by the Year 2000" in the 1970s and the evolution towards greater social accountability of medical schools called for by WHO in 1995.[20]

Training for Health Equity Network (THEnet) is a collaboration of schools of medicine and health sciences with a social accountability mandate. This has been defined by the schools themselves as an obligation to orient teaching, research, and service activities to addressing the priority health needs of the communities they have a mandate to serve, with a particular focus on the needs of underserved populations in their regions. They share a core mission to increase the number, quality, retention, and performance of health professionals in these communities.

Supported by The Atlantic Philanthropies, THEnet grew out of a project of the Global Health Education Consortium to identify innovative schools of medicine and health sciences addressing the health and social needs of underserved and marginalized populations. Eight schools of health sciences were identified. They are: Faculty of Health Sciences at Walter Sisulu University (WSU) in South Africa; Latin American School of Medicine in Cuba (ELAM); the Comprehensive Community Physician Training Program in Venezuela (CCPTP); Northern Ontario School of Medicine in Canada (NOSM); Flinders University School of Medicine and James Cook Faculty of Medicine, Health, and Molecular Sciences (JCU) in Australia; and Ateneo de Zamboanga University School of Medicine (ADZU) and the University of Philippines School of Health Sciences (SHS) in Leyte in the Philippines.

These institutions operate in highly diverse contexts. Current total enrollment in the schools ranges from 200 to 20,000 students. Training settings vary from remote indigenous communities in Canada and Australia, rural regions of Africa to urban slums in Venezuela, and marginalized communities in the Philippines, including conflict-ridden Mindanao.

Yet, these schools based in high- and low-income countries, shared common principles and strategies. As a starting point for their education, research, and service activities, the schools, in partnerships with key stakeholders, identify priority health and social needs of their reference populations, using a variety of instruments including epidemiologic and demographic tools, surveys, focus group discussions, and community workshops. The identification of needs is an essential step in defining graduate-desired competencies, guiding education, service programs, and prioritizing research activities **Fig. 1**.[21]

THEnet schools recruit and support students from communities with the greatest needs. All developed integrated primary care-oriented curricula in partnership with the communities they serve. The curricula are aligned with priority needs and delivered in primary, secondary, and tertiary care settings. The schools' pedagogical methodologies are student-centered, problem-oriented, and service-based. All recruit and train community-based practitioners as teachers and mentors, and faculty and programs emphasize and model commitment to public service.[22] Each school's leadership and faculty work closely with other health system actors with the aim of producing health workers with locally relevant competencies. What is more, these schools

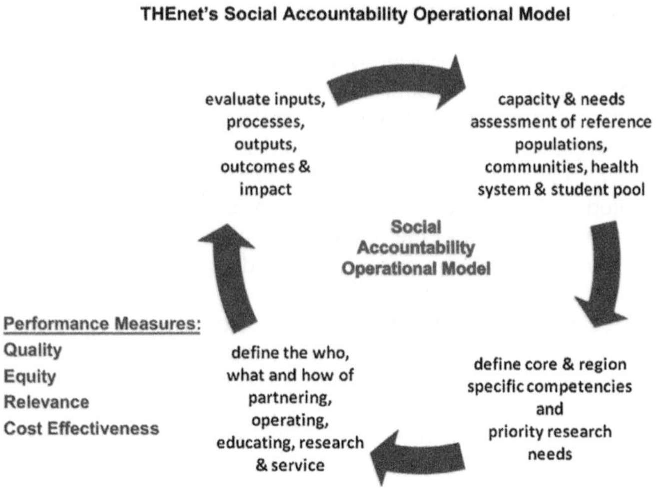

Fig. 1. The social accountability operational model.

hold themselves accountable for producing outcomes aligned with short- and long-term workforce and health system needs (**Box 1**).

THEnet schools, challenging prevailing orthodoxies, faced similar challenges and obstacles including institutional isolation and skepticism from more traditional medical schools. Some critics argue that rural and community-oriented medical schools sacrifice academic standards for example by recruiting students from rural and underserved areas. Evidence suggests otherwise. All member schools produce graduates with average or above average results on national examinations. For example, with

Box 1
Training for Health Equity Network schools common principles and strategies

- Health and social needs of targeted communities guide education, research, and service programs
- Students recruited from the communities with the greatest health care needs
- Programs are located within or in close proximity to the communities they serve
- Much of the learning takes place in the community instead of predominantly in university and hospital settings
- Curriculum integrates basic and clinical sciences with population health and social sciences, and early clinical contact increases the relevance and value of theoretical learning
- Pedagogical methodologies are student-centered, problem and service-based, and supported by information technology
- Community-based practitioners are recruited and trained as teachers and mentors
- Partnering with health system actors to produce locally relevant competencies
- Faculty and programs emphasize and model commitment to public service

average national passing rates of 50%, ADZU has a cumulative 90% passing rate at the national licensing examinations in the Philippines, and SHS medical graduates achieve passing rates above the national average. Both schools have had graduates among the nation's top 10.[23] In 2009, NOSM's first medical graduating class ranked first in clinical decision making on the Medical Council of Canada qualifying examinations. For overall performance, NOSM ranked 6th among Canada's 17 medical schools.[24] Out of 98 physicians from Flinders University Parallel Rural Community Curriculum who graduated between 1997 and 2005, 53% had chosen a rural career path.[25] The newly established medical schools at James Cook University identified similar trends in their 5 graduating cohorts. Of 350 graduates 70% did their 1st postgraduate year away from a major metropolitan hospital, and 53% of 1st year postgraduates selected regional or remote locations for their 2nd and 3rd year of training. Thus most postgraduates have chosen to general and rural practice where the needs are the greatest.[26]

Not only are the schools providing health services where access to services is limited or nonexistent, the schools in existence for more than 15 years also have impressive regional retention rates for their graduates. Of WSU graduates in the last 25 years, 80% are still working in the rural areas of Eastern Cape and Kwazulu Natal. In the Philippines, where 80% of physicians plan for an overseas career,[27] over a period of more than 20 years between 80% and 90% of SHS multiprofessional program students have stayed in their rural communities, depending on health worker category.[23] In the 15 years of ADZU's operations, the percentage of municipalities without doctors in ADZU's catchment area has dropped from 80% to 69%. More than 90% of its graduates have stayed in previously doctor-less areas, with 96% remaining in the Philippines. While research to account for confounding variables is not yet completed, infant mortality in the catchment area of the ADZU region has fallen from 75 to 80 deaths per 1000 live births to an impressive 8 deaths per 1000 live births.[28]

NETWORKING TO DEVELOP CAPACITY AND EVIDENCE

To leverage global learning on health workforce development and broaden and sustain the impact of global health investments, there is a need to strengthen the knowledge base on effective strategies to train, retain, and sustain health workers in neglected communities.[29]

Although documented outcomes and impact of socially accountable medical education show great promise, particularly in terms of retention of health workers, more rigorous, comprehensive, longitudinal studies are needed.[23,30,31]

Given THEnet schools' shared mission and similar strategies, they recognized the need to collaborate to systematically build a common evidence and knowledge base on a socially accountable health workforce. As a result, THEnet schools identified 3 important areas for collaboration: development and implementation of a common evaluation framework, cross-institutional research, and the creation of a community of practice.

A Common Evaluation Framework

Evidence on the impact of health professional education on population health and health systems is limited. Most evaluations of academic performance focus on input indicators (such as number and quality of faculty and facilities) or output indicators (eg, number of graduates, skills and knowledge learned, research published, and grants received).[32] Moreover, given that educational interventions occur in the dynamic and complex nature of health systems, the linear input-outcome-impact chains fail to explain how and why specific strategies and programs work and in what context.[33] Thus new evaluation tools are needed.[32,34]

In response, having agreed on the key components of social accountability in medical education, the THEnet schools developed and tested an evaluation framework to measure social accountability in practice. THEnet used the Boelen and Woollard's Social Accountability Conceptualization–Production–Usability model as the foundation.[15] The key questions in **Box 2** illustrate the core questions it seeks to answer.

The goal of the common framework is to create and pilot an agreed process, set of tools, measures, and standards for evaluating socially accountable health professions schools and to foster evidence-based health workforce education. For the core questions underlying the framework, see **Box 2**.

The framework was tested at 6 schools during 2010, reviewed, and modified based on feedback received. In 2011, it will be tested at several schools that are currently not members of THEnet. Testing the tool at different institutions provides opportunities to validate the instruments and increase their reliability and utilization in different contexts. The indicators identified may eventually form the basis for the development of new accreditation standards that provide evidence of a medical school's impact on the public good.

Although the focus of the framework initially was on medical education, it was developed in the context of health workforce development in general. This is but the first step in a broader process of developing tools that apply to other health professions. In fact several member schools are already training a range of health professional cadres, and some have tested the framework in other health disciplines.

Collaborative Research

While initiatives to scale up the global health workforce are mushrooming, there is a lack of cross-institutional research and systematic data collection of what works, how, and in what context. Aggregated evidence-based and context-based knowledge is needed to support and foster health education programs that meet health and health system needs.[4,32]

The ultimate goal of THEnet's research activities is to help health professions institutions design, manage, and evaluate education, research, and services programs that maximize their contribution to health equity and health system strengthening. For example, THEnet is developing a longitudinal research project to measure the impact of socially accountable medical education through the lens of graduate outcomes. To better understand how schools can affect change, this tracking project will use a systems lens to map out interconnected factors including actors, relationships, and processes that influence the career choices, practice location, and retention of health workers.

The testing of the evaluation framework at THEnet schools revealed that by mobilizing and empowering communities and other stakeholders and trying to engender commitment to serve in difficult environments, these frontline schools are involved in successful social change efforts. However, these efforts are not adequately documented, and more work is needed to capture, share, and harness the tacit knowledge and undocumented practices that have proved successful. Several research projects are planned to fill in this knowledge gap.

THEnet is a collaboration of schools in different stages of development—some new, others established; some have been innovative from inception, and others have changed from traditional approaches. Some schools are in high-income countries, and others are in low-income countries. Some schools operate in centralized systems, others in more open systems. This diversity also allows validating tools across

Box 2
Training for Health Equity Network's key questions for socially accountable health profession schools

Conceptualization: how does the school work?

1. What are the school's values, and how can they be operationalized?
2. Who are the populations and the health system the school is serving?
3. What are priority needs, and how can fulfillment of those needs be ensured?
4. Who should be collaborated with to have the impact being sought, and how do can these people be engaged?
5. Are patients, students, faculty, communities, health service providers, and health system actors being included when programs are planned, managed, and evaluated?
6. Are strategies and policies developed through collaboration with stakeholders, and does decision making involve meaningful participation from all stakeholders?

Production: what does the school do?

7. Does the education program reflect the priority health and social needs of the communities served, as defined by community partnerships, and is this is evident in programs and the services provided?
8. Do students learn in the context they are expected to work in, and do the placements provide adequate exposure to priority health needs and interprofessional exposure?
9. Do students reflect the demographics of the school's reference population, and do they have the background most likely to work and stay in areas where they are needed?
10. Is the school's research agenda based on priority health needs of its reference populations and the context in which the school operates, and are these needs developed and undertaken in partnership with key stakeholders?

Outcomes and impact: what difference is the school making?

11. Are research projects building knowledge that help meet priority health and health system needs? Are they contributing to decision making and informing or changing policies and practice?
12. What contributions is the school making to improve the quality, quantity, and equity of care in the populations it serves?
13. Where alumni working, and what are they doing?
14. Are the school's education interventions having the desired effect on the behavior and practice of its graduates?
15. Are strategies and decision-making processes having the desired long-term effect?
16. What difference has the school made to its reference population and health system?
17. How has the school shared ideas and influenced others?
18. How does the school engage in a continuous process of critical reflection and analysis with others?
19. Does the school influence policymakers, education providers, and other stakeholders to transform the health system to increase performance and health equity?
20. What impact has the school made with other schools?

context. It provides an opportunity for the development of rich case studies and comparative long-term cost–benefit analysis model to measure projected returns on investment in health profession institutions striving towards greater social accountability.

Community of Practice

THEnet initially started as a collaborative platform between 8 founding schools of health sciences and medicine. After an incubation period, THEnet's Community of Practice (CoP) is opening up to other health profession schools with institutional commitment towards social accountability. The CoP aims to offer a 1-stop shop for social accountability, offering instant access to resources, peers, potential research collaborators, and experts, with the overarching goal to strengthen institutional capacity. It provides a secure space for experimentation, learning, and cocreating of new knowledge and tools. It will be open to faculty, staff, and students of member schools, providing opportunities to learn, contribute ideas, reflect on experiences with others, access tools, and engage in a supportive peer network.

SUMMARY

Global health inequity is a key global policy concern.[35] Medically underserved communities suffer a high burden of morbidity and mortality, increasing with remoteness where access to health services is limited.[8] A major part of the problem is an overall shortage and maldistribution of the health workforce. Insufficient numbers, emphasis on specialist training rather than generalist practice, and the global brain drain towards high-income urban centers are just some of the issues facing the medically underserved. Yet, despite their key role in health system development, few health profession schools, responsible for producing the health workforce and research systems needs, define themselves in terms of this role. Institutions are rarely held accountable for producing outcomes aligned with priority health workforce and health system needs. There is a lack of understanding of how these institutions can optimize their contribution to health equity and health system strengthening.

A new international collaborative of health professions schools with a core mission to meet the needs of underserved populations, THEnet, was recently created. THEnet is developing and disseminating evidence, challenging assumptions, and developing tools that support health profession institutions striving to be more responsive to societies' changing needs. It is evolving common evaluation tools, conducting transdisciplinary and cross-institutional research, and developing a knowledge base as well as an action-oriented CoP.

Health profession institutions should be effective partners in health system development. More research is needed to understand how institutions in high and low resources settings can better address the health and social needs of the population and region they serve and how they become catalysts for social change. When schools of medicine and health sciences cross disciplines, use their commonalities and differences to support each other, reflect on specific practice oriented topics, cocreate and utilize knowledge and tools, then institutional capacity grows. As a result, the return on investment in global health is multiplied as schools around the globe gain the capacity to scan globally and reinvent locally.

REFERENCES

1. Tomson G. The impact of global processes on health systems in Europe. Global Health Europe research paper number 2. Geneva (Switzerland): Global Health Europe; 2010.
2. Lu C, Schneider MT, Gubbins P, et al. Public financing of health in developing countries: a cross-national systematic analysis. Lancet 2010;375(9723):1375–87.

3. Ravishankar N, Gubbins P, Cooley RJ, et al. Financing of global health: tracking development assistance for health from 1990 to 2007. Lancet 2009;373(9681): 2113–24.
4. Frenk J, Chen L, Bhutta Z, et al. Health professionals for a new century: transforming education to strengthen health systems in an interdependent world. Lancet 2010;376(9756):1923–58.
5. Anand S, Bärnighausen T. Human resources and health outcomes: cross-country econometric study. Lancet 2004;364(9445):1603–9.
6. Chen L, Evans T, Anand S, et al. Human resources for health: overcoming the crisis. Lancet 2004;364(9449):1984–90.
7. Anyangwe SC, Mtonga C. Inequities in the global health workforce: the greatest impediment to health in sub-Saharan Africa. Int J Environ Res Public Health 2007; 4(2):93–100.
8. Dussault G, Franceschini MC. Not enough there, too many here: understanding geographical imbalances in the distribution of the health workforce. Hum Resour Health 2006;4:12.
9. Health Resources and Services Administration. Shortage designation: HPSAs, MUAs, & MUPs. Washington, DC: US Department of Health and Human Services; 2009.
10. Rieselbach R, Crouse BJ, Frohna JG. Teaching primary care in community health centers: addressing the workforce crisis for the underserved. Ann Intern Med 2010;152:118–22.
11. Chen L, Boufford JI. Fatal flows-doctors on the move. N Engl J Med 2005;353: 1850–2.
12. Mullan F, Frehywot S, Omaswa F, et al. Medical schools in sub-Saharan Africa. Lancet 2011;377(9771):1113–21.
13. Institute of Medicine. Health professions education: a bridge to quality. Washington, DC: National Academy Press; 2003. p. 1.
14. Cooke M, Irby DM, O'Brian BC. A summary of educating physicians: a call for reform of medical school and residency. Stanford (CA): The Carnegie Foundation for the Advancement of Teaching; 2010.
15. Boelen C, Woollard RF. Social accountability and accreditation: a new frontier for educational institutions. Med Educ 2009;43:887–94.
16. van Zanten M, Norcini JJ, Boulet JR, et al. Overview of accreditation of undergraduate medical education programmes worldwide. Med Educ 2008;42:930–7.
17. Horton R. A new epoch for health professionals' education. Lancet 2010; 376(9756):1875–7.
18. Menand L. The marketplace of ideas: reform and resistance in the American university. New York: Norton; 2010.
19. Skochelak SA. Decade of reports calling for change in medical education: what do they say? Acad Med 2010;85(9):S26–33.
20. World Health Organization. Reorienting medical education and medical practice for health for all. World health assembly resolution WHA48.8. Geneva (Switzerland): World Health Organization; 1995.
21. Palsdottir B, Neusy AJ, Reed G. Building the evidence base: networking innovative socially accountable medical education programmes. Educ Health 2008;21(2):177.
22. Strasser R, Neusy AJ. Context counts: training health workers in and for rural and remote areas. Bull World Health Organ 2010;88:777–82.
23. Siega-Sur JL. The UPM-SHS: where health workers are trained to stay and serve. Available at: http://www.up.edu.ph/upforum.php?i=97&archive=yes&yr=2005&mn=7. Accessed September 20, 2010.

24. Larkin K. NOSM's Charter Class Students Score Above National Average on Medical Council of Canada Examinations. NOSM Web site. Available at: http://www.nosm.ca/about_us/media_room/media_releases/media_release.aspx?id59592. Accessed November 10, 2010.
25. Stagg P, Greenhhill J, Worley PS. A new model to understand career choice. Rural Remote Health 2009;9:1245.
26. Sen Gupta TK, Hays R, Murray RB. Intern choices for James Cook University graduates [letter]. Med J Aust 2007;187(3):197.
27. Cheng MH. The Philippines' health worker exodus. Lancet 2009;373(9658): 111–2.
28. Cristobal F, Concepcion P, Samson R. Responding to the clarion call to health for more. Poster presented at Social Accountability in the African Context. Walter Sisulu University, Mthatha, South Africa, October 7–9, 2010.
29. World Health Organization. The World health report 2006: working together for health. Geneva (Switzerland): World Health Organization; 2006.
30. Worley P, Martin A, Prideaux D, et al. Vocational career paths of graduate entry medical students at Flinders University: a comparison of rural, remote and tertiary tracks. Med J Aust 2008;188(3):177–8.
31. Christobal L, Kreutz W. Medical Education For Health Development: Perspectives from the New Zamboanga medical school Republic of the Philippines. The Meducator 2001;1(1).
32. Palsdottir B. Institutional development for Africa—towards greater accountability for results in return on investment: the long-term impact of building health care capacity in Africa. Washington, DC: Accordia Global Health Foundation; 2010. p. 43–50.
33. de Savigny D, Adams T. Systems thinking for health systems strengthening: alliance for health policy and systems research. Geneva (Switzerland): World Health Organization; 2009.
34. Zurn P, Dal Poz MR, Stilwell B, et al. Imbalance in the health workforce. Hum Resour Health 2004;2:13.
35. Labonté R, Gagnon ML. Framing health and foreign policy: lessons for global health diplomacy. Global Health 2010;6:14.

Teaching the Basics: Core Competencies in Global Health

Megan A.M. Arthur, MSc[a], Robert Battat[b],
Timothy F. Brewer, MD, MPH[c,*]

KEYWORDS

• Medical education • Global health • Core Competencies

WHAT IS GLOBAL HEALTH?

Global health has been defined as "...the goal of improving health for all people by reducing avoidable diseases, disabilities, and deaths"[1] and an "area for study, research, and practice that places a priority on improving health and achieving equity in health for all people worldwide".[2] These definitions highlight the multinational, multidisciplinary, and equity-oriented nature of this emerging field. Global health involves social, political, economic, and environmental considerations that affect the health of communities and individuals around the world. Yet the same interconnectedness that facilitates the globalization of diseases is also manifested through the unprecedented interaction and cooperation between governments, civil society organizations, and individuals across time zones and borders to address health issues. Examples of this cooperation include large-scale multinational health efforts such as the United Nations Millennium Development Goals or the US President's Emergency Program for AIDS Relief.[3] Technological advances that permit instant knowledge sharing around the world, creating the capacity to transform medical education and care, are also rapidly evolving. The problem is therefore linked to the solution. Globalization has produced new multidisciplinary multinational health challenges, and the global

Funding support: The Core Competencies project was funded in part by a grant from the Donner Canadian Foundation. The funding organization did not play any role in the design and conduct of the study; the collection, management, analysis, and interpretation of the data; or the preparation, review, or approval of this article.
Conflict of interest: The authors have no conflicts to disclose.
[a] Global Health Programs, Faculty of Medicine, McGill University, Purvis Hall, Room 41, 1020 Pine Avenue West, Montreal, QC H31 1A2, Canada
[b] Faculty of Medicine, McGill University, 3655 Promenade Sir William Osler, Montreal, Quebec H3G 1Y6, Canada
[c] Global Health Programs, Faculty of Medicine, McGill University, Purvis Hall, Room 42, 1020 Pine Avenue West, Montreal, QC H31 1A2, Canada
* Corresponding author.
E-mail address: timothy.brewer@mail.mcgill.ca

Infect Dis Clin N Am 25 (2011) 347–358
doi:10.1016/j.idc.2011.02.013
id.theclinics.com

health issues of the modern world require coordinated multisectoral, multidisciplinary, and multinational efforts to achieve effective resolutions.

GLOBAL HEALTH TRAINING IN MEDICAL SCHOOLS: NEED AND CURRENT STATE

Medical education is increasingly being pushed to adapt, internally by the explosive growth in scientific knowledge and externally by rapid transformations in the global context. In response, experts are rethinking the approach to and content of medical education for the twenty-first century, including the role for global health.[4] Reasons to include global health training as part of routine medical education include, among others, the tremendous increase in student and faculty interest, the growing percentage of immigrants in the United States and Canadian domestic populations, the rapid spread of communicable diseases by international travel, and the need for all physicians to have basic knowledge of major factors affecting health and the delivery of health care.[3] Global health provides a framework to address issues such as inequities in health, cultural competency, globalization of health care, and social and environmental determinants of health crucial to modern medical education.

Although the need for global health curricular content is increasingly recognized, there has been a paucity of research examining the development of global health content for medical curricula.[5] In general, the literature reflects a fragmented and insufficient response on the part of medical schools to the increased student demand for global health content.[6,7] Much of the literature to date regarding global health medical education focuses on international electives or activities at individual medical schools.[8,9] A survey of global health training in Canadian medical schools in 2006 found that global health content was haphazard and lacking in uniform objectives or guidelines.[5] The lack of coordination in curricular development has resulted in wide variations between medical schools in the type, quantity, and quality of global health content offered. Where global health components are provided, there are variations in the format and content of global health materials, the year in which it is taught, whether the courses are required or elective, and whether they are didactic or experiential.[5]

While variations in educational approaches are an important source of innovation, the lack of consensus that characterizes contemporary global health training may have detrimental consequences. In the absence of formal learning opportunities, medical students are pursuing their own programs and electives in global health, often with little or no faculty oversight.[5] This situation presents the risk of students practicing beyond their competency level, which may lead to harm for patients, themselves, and the educational and clinical institutions in which they study.[10]

Beyond the clinical aspects, medical graduates lacking appropriate global health training will be unprepared to recognize and meet the challenges of an increasingly interdependent world and the needs of the patients and populations they will serve.[3] Coordinating the development of medical education systems for a new global context of medical care requires a systematic approach supported by key organizations and accreditation bodies.[5] The lack of consensus among schools and leaders regarding what constitutes fundamental elements in global health training must be addressed in order to counter the fragmentation and inconsistency of current pedagogical approaches.[3,5] One step in this process is to seek consensus regarding the core competencies that all medical students, regardless of their interest in global health, should possess before graduating. Although particular themes have been identified in the literature,[7,11] a common set of criteria will help to ensure that all medical students receive appropriate and comparable global health training.

CREATING CORE COMPETENCIES IN GLOBAL HEALTH

To develop common standards for global health training in US and Canadian medical schools, the Global Health Education Consortium (GHEC) and the Association of Faculties of Medicine (AFMC) of Canada's Global Health Resource Group (GHRG) initiated a project to develop global health core curriculum guidelines appropriate for all medical students.[3] A literature review was conducted to assess the state of the knowledge regarding global health competencies for undergraduate medical education. This review identified 32 relevant articles; 11 retrieved articles described curricular competencies including the global burden of disease, travel medicine, health care disparities between countries, immigrant health, primary care within diverse cultural settings, and skills to better interface with different populations, cultures, and health care systems. Whereas each of these topics was mentioned in more than 1 article, no single topic was discussed in more than 5 of the reviewed articles, suggesting a lack of consensus within the literature regarding the essential global health competencies for medical students. The review also highlighted variations in the educational approaches used to teach these competencies.

Based on this review, a separate review of existing global health program websites, and expert opinion, the Committee developed a list of core competencies in global health for general medical education. In addition, the Committee detailed the essential knowledge and skills required within each competency topic area. These suggestions were then submitted for peer review to global health experts, medical educators, and students. Using a modified Delphi method, the Committee has developed recommendations outlining 7 topic areas and 18 competencies thought to be appropriate for global health training for all medical students. These recommendations are summarized in the following sections and in **Table 1**.

Global Burden of Disease

A basic understanding of the global burden of disease is an essential part of modern medical education. This knowledge is crucial for physicians to be informed participants in discussions of priority setting and the allocation of funds for health-related activities. Medical students should have a basic understanding of how morbidity and mortality are measured for health program monitoring, what the major causes of morbidity and mortality around the globe are, and how disease risk varies by world region. This includes understanding the major categories of morbidity and mortality used by the World Health Organization (WHO) and how they vary between high-, middle-, and low-income regions. Students should also have familiarity with major public health efforts to reduce health disparities globally, such as the Millennium Development Goals; they should be able to identify a health objective from the Millennium Development Goals and to describe the function and role of the WHO in developing health care policies. Finally, medical graduates should be able to demonstrate familiarity with health care funding mechanisms, priority-setting, and funding for health-related research, as well as be able to describe challenges to the existing health care system in their region.

Health Implications of Travel, Migration, and Displacement

The proper management of patients necessitates taking into consideration varying perspectives and implications due to international travel, foreign birth, or differing cultural backgrounds. Over the past several decades, economic and social globalization, particularly through migration, has led to changing social landscapes in nations around the world. The range of health concerns experienced by migrants and travelers

Table 1
Global health essential core competencies for medical students

Topic Area	Competency Description
1. Global burden of disease	1. Knowledge of the major global causes of morbidity and mortality and how health risks vary by gender and income across regions a. To demonstrate competency in this area, students should: i. Be able to describe the principle measures of morbidity and mortality and their roles and limitations for health program monitoring, evaluation and priority setting. This will involve the ability to: 1. Describe the concepts of under 5 mortality rate, life expectancy, quality adjusted life-year (QALY) and disability adjusted life-year (DALY) 2. Explain how life expectancy, QALY and DALY may be used to make general health comparisons within and/or between countries and regions 3. Identify changes in under 5 mortality as the major reason for changes in life expectancy ii. Be able to identify the major categories of morbidity and mortality used by the World Health Organization (WHO) and to describe how the relative importance of each category, and of the leading diagnoses within each category, vary by age, gender, WHO region, and between high, middle and low-income regions. For example: 1. Communicable and parasitic diseases, maternal, perinatal and childhood conditions, and nutritional deficiencies are more significant causes of morbidity and mortality in low-income regions 2. Non-communicable conditions are important and of increasing significance in high, middle and low-income regions 3. Injuries are a more important cause of morbidity and mortality in middle and low-income regions iii. Be able to efficiently access global health data from sources such as the WHO Global Burden of Disease measures and understand the limitations of these data 2. Be able to knowledgeably discuss priority setting, healthcare rationing and funding for health and health-related research b. To demonstrate competency in this area, students should: i. Be familiar with the concepts of priority setting and healthcare rationing and be able to describe challenges for the existing healthcare system in your community/country, such as: 1. Lack of health insurance for a substantial proportion of the population; 2. Waiting times for elective procedures and the public/private balance for healthcare; 3. Unequal distribution of physicians between urban and rural areas and between primary care and sub-specialty fields ii. Be aware of global systems of funding for health research and service provision and describe what is meant by the concept of neglected diseases
2. Health implications of travel, migration and displacement	1. Understand health risks associated with travel, with emphasis on potential risks and appropriate management, including referrals a. To demonstrate competency in this area, students should: i. Know general patterns of disease and injury in various world regions, and how to counsel or refer patients traveling to or returning from those areas ii. Understand the importance of a recent or past travel history when patients present for care and have proficiency in obtaining a relevant travel history iii. Recognize potentially serious or life threatening conditions such as the febrile traveler and be able to arrange timely, appropriate referral

	2. Understand how travel and trade contribute to the spread of communicable diseases b. To demonstrate competency in this area, students should: i. Describe the concept of a pandemic and how global commerce and travel contribute to the spread of pandemics ii. Understand how travelers may contribute to outbreaks of communicable diseases such as measles in a context of local and international populations with varying levels of immunization iii. Be aware of the utility and limitations of common infection control and public health measures in dealing with local or global outbreaks 1. Examples include contact precautions, vaccinations, health advisories, prophylaxis, quarantines, isolation and travel restrictions iv. Know how to liaise with local or regional public health authorities and be aware of national and international public health organizations responsible for issuing health advisory recommendations 3. Understand the health risks related to migration, with emphasis on the potential risks and appropriate resources c. To demonstrate competency in this area, students should: i. Understand the basic demographics of foreign-born individuals in one's local community and country ii. Recognize when foreign birth places a patient at risk for unusual diseases or unusual presentation of injuries, common diseases or tropical diseases and make an appropriate diagnosis or referral iii. Be able to elicit individual health concerns in a culturally sensitive manner iv. Be familiar with issues that arise when communicating with patients and families using an interpreter
3. A) Social and economic determinants of health	1. Understand the relationship between health and social determinants of health, and how these vary across world regions a. To demonstrate competency in this area, students should: i. Define health inequity and be able to describe one local and one international example ii. List major social determinants of health and their impact on differences in life expectancy, major causes of morbidity and mortality and access to healthcare between and within countries 1. Topics include absolute and relative poverty, urbanization, crowding, inadequate housing, education (especially for females), gender and other inequities and discrimination based on race, ethnicity or other social determinants. iii. Be aware of local, national or international interventions to address health determinants 1. Examples include the UN Millennium Development Goals or the US Global Health Initiative
3. B) Population, resources and the environment	1. Understand the impact of rapid population growth and of unsustainable and inequitable resource consumption on important resources essential to human health, including water, sanitation and food supply, and know how these resources vary across world regions a. To demonstrate competency in this area, students should: i. Have a basic understanding regarding the adequacy of nutrition, potable water and sanitation in different regions around the world

(*continued on next page*)

Table 1
(continued)

Topic Area	Competency Description
	2. Describe the relationship between access to clean water, sanitation and nutrition on individual and population health b. To demonstrate competency in this area, students should: i. Explain the basic relationship between the availability of adequate nutrition, potable water and sanitation and risk of communicable and chronic diseases and provide specific examples 1. Appropriate topics include the interactions between protein, caloric, and micronutrient malnutrition and various major diseases; and the interactions between inadequate clean water supplies and good sanitation and diarrheal and parasitic diseases 3. Describe the relationship between environmental degradation, pollution and health c. To demonstrate competency in this area, students should: i. Be able to explain examples of causes of pollution and environmental degradation and their consequences for health globally. For example: 1. The effects of air pollution on chronic lung and cardiovascular disease 2. The relationship between environmental pollution and cancers i. Radon and lung cancer; benzene and leukemia
4. Globalization of health and healthcare	1. Understand how global trends in healthcare practice, commerce and culture contribute to health and the quality and availability of healthcare locally and internationally a. To demonstrate competency in this area, students should: i. Describe different national models for public and/or private provision of healthcare and their impact on the health of the population and individuals ii. Be aware of examples of how globalization and trade including trade agreements affect availability of healthcare such as patented or essential medicines 2. Be familiar with major multinational efforts to improve health globally b. To demonstrate competency in this area, students should: i. Describe the core functions and role of the WHO in developing healthcare policies and practices ii. Discuss the function/intention of the Millennium Development Goals and identify health-related objectives, including: 1. Reduce child mortality 2. Improve maternal health 3. Eradicate extreme poverty and hunger 4. Combat HIV/AIDS, malaria and other diseases 3. Understand and describe general trends and influences in the global availability and movement of healthcare workers c. To demonstrate competency in this area, students should: i. Know the approximate extent of national and global healthcare worker availability (shortage) ii. Describe the most common patterns of healthcare worker migration ("brain drain") and its impact on healthcare availability in both the country that the healthcare worker leaves and the country to which he/she migrates

5. Healthcare in low-resource settings	1. Identify barriers to health and healthcare in low-resource settings locally and internationally a. To demonstrate competency in this area, students should: i. Describe barriers to recruitment, training and retention of human resources in underserved areas such as rural, inner-city and indigenous communities within high- and low-income countries ii. Describe the effect of distance and inadequate infrastructure on the delivery of healthcare 1. For example, be able to discuss the effects of travel costs, poor roads, lack of mailing address or phone system, lack of medicines, inadequate staffing, and inadequate and unreliable laboratory and diagnostic support iii. Identify barriers to appropriate prevention and treatment programs in low-resource settings 1. For example, be able to discuss the effects of low literacy and health literacy, user fees, lack of health insurance, costs of medicines and treatments, therapies and procedures, advanced presentation of disease, lack of provider access to management guidelines and training including continuing professional development, concerns regarding quality of care–real or perceived, cultural barriers to care, underutilization of existing resources, issues facing scaling up and implementation of successful programs 2. Demonstrate an understanding of healthcare delivery strategies in low-resource settings, especially the role of community-based healthcare and primary care models b. To demonstrate competency in this area, students should: i. Differentiate between and highlight the benefits and disadvantages of horizontal and vertical implementation strategies ii. Be familiar with the concept of an essential medicines list and understand its role in ensuring access to standardized, effective treatments 3. Demonstrate an understanding of cultural and ethical issues in working with underserved populations c. To demonstrate competency in this area, students should: i. Discuss the professional and ethical issues involved in allowing trainees to practice or assist in settings where they may be perceived and treated as healthcare workers, even by local healthcare providers 1. Explain the student's professional and ethical responsibilities in resource-poor settings 2. For example, be able to discuss the impact on local staff, patient perceptions and risks to patients and students 4. Demonstrate the ability to adapt clinical skills and practice in a resource-constrained setting d. To demonstrate competency in this area, students should: i. Identify signs and symptoms for common major diseases that facilitate diagnosis in the absence of advanced testing often unavailable in low-resource settings 1. For example, HIV/AIDS, TB, malaria, childhood pneumonia, cardiovascular disease, cancer, diabetes ii. Describe clinical interventions and integrated strategies that have been demonstrated to substantially improve individual and/or population health in low-resource settings 1. For example, be able to discuss immunizations, an essential drugs list, maternal, child and family planning health programs

(*continued on next page*)

Table 1
(continued)

Topic Area	Competency Description
	5. For students who participate in electives in low-resource settings outside their home situations, demonstrate that they have participated in training to prepare for this elective e. To demonstrate competency in this area, students should: i. Demonstrate preparation in the following areas: 1. Personal health: basic health precautions, immunizations, health insurance, personal protective equipment, post exposure prophylaxis for HIV, access to medical care 2. Travel safety: orientation upon arrival, packing requirements, registering at home embassy, travel advisory warnings, emergency preparedness 3. Cultural awareness: basic understanding of culture (especially as it pertains to health), intercultural relationships, gender, family and community roles, and religion 4. Language competencies: language basics, host language expectations and availability of interpreters 5. Ethical considerations: evaluate motivations for participating in international elective, discuss potential ethical dilemmas prior to departure, code of conduct, appropriate licensing, local mentor/supervision, communications, and patient privacy 6. Review guidelines for professionalism in electronic communications such as blogging, emails, and/or distribution of photographs taken in low resource settings 7. Understand the possible historical and current socio-political and economical factors pertaining to the region in which they will work and how these may affect their work abroad
6. Human rights in global health	1. Demonstrate a basic understanding of the relationship between health and human rights a. To demonstrate competency in this area, students should: i. Have an understanding of the right to health and how this right is defined under international agreements such as the United Nations' Universal Declaration of Human Rights or the Declaration of Alma-Ata ii. Discuss how social, economic, political or cultural factors may affect an individual's or community's right to healthcare 1. Examples include availability, accessibility, affordability and quality

These recommendations represent their authors' opinion and should not be considered as representing the opinion of the AFMC.

Abbreviations: DALY, disability-adjusted life-year; HIV, human immunodeficiency virus; QALY, quality-adjusted life-year; TB, tuberculosis; UN, United Nations; WHO, World Health Organization.

From an AFMC Resource Group on Global Health/GHEC joint committee; with permission.

requires that domestic health care professionals be well trained in a broader range of health issues to meet the needs of increasingly multicultural and diverse populations. This training includes competency in cross-cultural communication and interactions.

In 2004, 763 million people crossed international borders.[12] Each year, up to 8% of travelers seek health care while abroad or upon returning home.[13] Although travel medicine has emerged to accommodate the need for expertise in providing pre-travel and post-travel advice,[14] all physicians should know how to take a basic travel history and when to refer or treat individuals with possible travel-related illnesses. Health professionals also require some understanding of how the global economy and travel contribute to the spread of communicable diseases, such as the severe acute respiratory syndrome epidemic of 2003 or the H1N1 pandemic of 2009. These experiences demonstrate the undeniable link between global and domestic health systems, the need for training in public health practice, and the need to better comprehend the medical risks of an interconnected world.

Social and Economic Determinants of Health

Dramatic inequities in health status exist within and between countries. According to the WHO Commission on Social Determinants of Health, "These inequities in health... arise because of the circumstances in which people grow, live, work, and age, and the systems put in place to deal with illness. The conditions in which people live and die are, in turn, shaped by political, social, and economic forces".[15] Morbidity and mortality vary according to social determinants, including education, occupation, income, social class, gender, age, and ethnicity, among others. Consistently, a lower socioeconomic status is associated with poorer health. Physicians should understand how social and economic conditions affect health, both to recognize disease risk factors in their patients and to contribute to improving public health.

Global health strives to achieve health equity for all. Medical education has a crucial responsibility to cultivate health professionals who embrace their role as advocates for the promotion of population health and the provision of effective health care services. Integral to the professional role of physicians within society are the values of altruism and compassion[16] and the need to address issues of social justice and inequities in access to health care.[17,18] Major medical organizations and licensing bodies have recognized this role and emphasized that addressing health care inequalities within and beyond domestic borders is a fundamental principle of physician professionalism.[17,19] In order to cultivate in future physicians the characteristics required to meet the needs of contemporary societies and the expectations of professional organizations, medical schools should incorporate social and economic determinants of health learning objectives as integral components of their educational programs.

Population, Resources, and the Environment

Demographic projections anticipate that the world's population will increase by 40% by 2050, with almost all of this expansion occurring in low-income countries. This growth could have a major adverse impact on the availability of food, water, and other essential resources, as well as exacerbate pollution. Medical students should have an understanding of the health impacts of rapid population growth and unsustainable and inequitable consumption of essential resources, including water and food supply. Students should also be aware of regional variation in access to these resources and the effects of inequitable consumption on individuals and communities around the world. They should be able to describe the relationship between access to clean water, sanitation, and nutrition to individual and population health.

Globalization of Health and Health Care

Globalization affects all aspects of health care, including the ability of governments or organizations to provide adequate care, the evolution of the local health care system, disease patterns, and the movement of health care workers within a global shortage of health human resources. Medical students should be able to understand and describe general trends in and influences on the global availability and movement of health care workers, as well as know how global trends in health care practice, commerce, and culture contribute to health and the quality and availability of health care locally and internationally.

Health Care in Low-Resource Settings

Health systems in low-resource settings often differ from those in the high-resource urban environments in which medical students are typically trained. Low-resource settings, including those among marginalized populations and rural environments in high-income countries, often face considerable human resource shortages within health care, as well as broader infrastructural inadequacies and barriers to prevention and treatment programs. These barriers may include inadequate local health system infrastructures; poor public infrastructure such as roads, schools, and telecommunications; cultural and linguistic barriers; low literacy rates; lack of health insurance; costs of medicines and therapies; advanced presentation of disease; lack of provider access to continuing education; and underutilization of available resources. Medical students should be aware of the realities of health care delivery in resource-poor settings and standards of clinical appropriateness in different environments. Further, students who travel abroad to participate in elective programs in low-resource settings should receive appropriate specialized orientation and training. This training should include such topics as personal health, travel safety, and ethical challenges that they may encounter, as well as competency with respect to the historical, sociopolitical, cultural, and linguistic contexts in which they will be learning.

Besides specific training in working within low-resource settings, medical graduates should be able to demonstrate an understanding of how primary health care delivery strategies may reduce health inequalities through programs such as universal and equitable access to health services, immunization programs, essential medicines lists, maternal and child health programs, community health worker programs, and primary care as a focal point and coordinating mechanism for comprehensive health service provision at all levels.[20]

Human Rights in Global Health

In 1948, the Universal Declaration of Human Rights established the right of every human being to enjoy a standard of living that promotes health and ensures adequate access to medical care.[21] However, despite the international community's agreement to health as a basic human right, health inequalities within and among nations persist and in many cases are widening. Future physicians should have an understanding of the intersection between health and human rights and how social, economic, political, and cultural factors affect individual and community rights to health care.

FUTURE DEVELOPMENTS

Compelling moral, ethical, professional, pedagogical, and economic imperatives support the integration of global health topics within medical school curriculum. Although the process of integrating global health into medical education is well underway at some medical schools, there remain substantial challenges to initiating global health training in others. As a new field, faculties and schools may benefit from resources and guidance to develop global health modules and teaching materials. The GHEC/AFMC GHRG core competencies project was undertaken with the goal of providing guidance for those programs interested in adding global health content to their curricula. In addition, it is hoped that these recommendations will stimulate discussion among medical educators, students, professional educational organizations, and accreditation bodies regarding global health training in medical education to facilitate consensus on necessary competencies for students. Through the use of the proposed set of core competencies established by this project, it is hoped that this model will be shared among medical educators and programs in an effort to build a coordinated approach to global health in medical education.

ACKNOWLEDGMENTS

The authors acknowledge the work of the Association of Faculties of Medicine of Canada Resource Group on Global Health/Global Health Education Consortium Joint Committee in developing the proposed competency guidelines. Committee members include Kelly Anderson, Timothy Brewer (Chair), Thuy Bui, Veronic Clair, Thomas Hall, Laura Janneck, Renee King, Anne McCarthy, Neal Nathanson, Sujal Parikh, Calvin Wilson, and Karen Yeates. The Committee was aided in its review of existing global health literature by Robert Battat, Gillian Seidman, Nicholas Chadi, Mohammed Yaameen Chanda, Jessica Nehme, Jennifer Hulme, Annie Li, and Nazlie Faridi. Winnie Chan also contributed to the collection of feedback on the drafted core competencies from the global health community.

REFERENCES

1. Institute of Medicine. The US commitment to global health: recommendations for the new administration. Washington, DC: National Academy Press; 2009.
2. Koplan JP, Bond TC, Merson MH, et al. Towards a common definition of global health. Lancet 2009;373(9679):1993–5.
3. Brewer TF, Saba N, Clair V. From boutique to basic: a call for standardised medical education in global health. Med Educ 2009;43(10):930–3.
4. Bhutta ZA, Chen L, Cohen J, et al. Education of health professionals for the 21st century: a global independent Commission. Lancet 2010;375(9721):1137–8.
5. Izadnegahdar R, Correia S, Ohata B, et al. Global health in Canadian medical education: current practices and opportunities. Acad Med 2008;83(2):192–8.
6. Drain PK, Primack A, Hunt DD, et al. Global health in medical education: a call for more training and opportunities. Acad Med 2007;82(3):226–30.
7. Houpt ER, Pearson RD, Hall TL. Three domains of competency in global health education: recommendations for all medical students. Acad Med 2007;82(3):222–5.
8. Heck JE, Wedemeyer D. International health education in US medical schools: trends in curriculum focus, student interest, and funding sources. Fam Med 1995;27(10):636–40.
9. Thompson MJ, Huntington MK, Hunt DD, et al. Educational effects of international health electives on U.S. and Canadian medical students and residents: a literature review. Acad Med 2003;78(3):342–7.
10. Banatvala N, Doyal L. Knowing when to say "no" on the student elective. Students going on electives abroad need clinical guidelines. BMJ 1998;316(7142):1404–5.
11. Evert J, Mautner D, Hoffman I. Developing global health curricula: a guidebook for US medical schools. In: Hall T, editor. Global health education consortium. San Francisco: GHEC; 2006. p. 32–8.

12. Hill DR. The burden of illness in international travelers. N Engl J Med 2006; 354(2):115–7.
13. Freedman DO, Weld LH, Kozarsky PE, et al. Spectrum of disease and relation to place of exposure among ill returned travelers. N Engl J Med 2006;354(2): 119–30.
14. Hill DR, Bia FJ. Coming of age in travel medicine and tropical diseases: a need for continued advocacy and mentorship. Infect Dis Clin North Am 2005;19(1): xv–xxi.
15. World Health Organization Commission on Social Determinants of Health. Closing the gap in a generation: health equity through action on the social determinants of health. Geneva (Switzerland): WHO Press; 2008.
16. Swick HM. Toward a normative definition of medical professionalism. Acad Med 2000;75(6):612–6.
17. American Board of Internal Medicine, American College of Physicians-American Society of Internal Medicine, European Federation of Internal Medicine. Medical professionalism in the new millennium: a physician charter. Ann Intern Med 2002; 136:243–6.
18. Frank JR, editor. Royal College of Physicians and Surgeons of Canada. The CanMEDS 2005 Physician Competency Framework. Ottawa Ontario Canada; 2005.
19. Code of Ethics. Ottawa Ontario Canada: Canadian Medical Association; 2004.
20. World Health Organization. The world health report 2008-primary health care (now more than ever). Geneva (Switzerland): WHO Press; 2008.
21. Section 25 Universal Declaration of Human Rights. Resolution 217 A (III). General Assembly of the United Nations; 1948.

Global Health Capacity and Workforce Development: Turning the World Upside Down

Lord Nigel Crisp, MA

KEYWORDS

• Global health • Health workforce • Codevelopment

Throughout this article the author distinguishes between *International Health* as a description which has traditionally been used in talking about the health of others—of people and peoples in countries other than our own—and the concept of *Global Health*, which embraces all those aspects of health shared by us all around the world. There are many of these shared concerns, as we shall see, from global pandemics to climate change and the availability of medicines, and together they reveal how interdependent we all are now in terms of our health.

This article discusses the vital importance to us all of building up the health workforce globally—as just such an example of this interdependence—and argue, further, that those of us living in the richer and more powerful countries of the world have a great deal to learn from people in low-income and middle-income countries who, without our resources and our baggage of history and vested interests, are innovating and developing new ways of tackling the spread of disease and improving health. We need, as argued by the author in the book *Turning the World Upside Down*,[1] to set aside our inbuilt assumptions and unconscious prejudices and see the world differently. We are dependent on each other and we can learn from each other.

INTERDEPENDENCE

Our most obvious interdependence is our shared vulnerability to infectious diseases and the ease with which these can now be transmitted around the world. In the fourteenth century the Black Death took 3 winters to cross Europe, in this century SARS

Lord Crisp is an independent member of the UK House of Lords, Honorary Professor at the London School of Hygiene and Tropical Medicine, Senior Fellow of the Institute for Healthcare Improvement, Distinguished Visiting Fellow at Harvard school of Public Health, and Honorary Fellow of St John's College, Cambridge.
The author has nothing to disclose.
The House of Lords, London SW1A 0PW, UK
E-mail address: crisp@parliament.uk

Infect Dis Clin N Am 25 (2011) 359–367
doi:10.1016/j.idc.2011.02.010
id.theclinics.com

(severe acute respiratory syndrome) took 3 days to spread across continents. We are all at risk and therefore, one might think, must fight such diseases together. However experience and the emergence of new diseases have shown us that this isn't at all as straightforward as it might seem. Our shared vulnerability has brought into focus issues of equity and rights.

Globally we need to share our knowledge; this also means sharing the tissues and specimens from ill and deceased people from which we can develop vaccines and treatments. However, as we have seen from recent cases, countries may not be willing to share such materials from their people if they do not believe that their citizens will share in the benefits of the drugs or vaccines developed from them. There is a real and understandable concern that these drugs or vaccines will only be available and affordable in the richer countries and that poorer countries will not get their share of the payback from a joint endeavor. The behavior of governments in both poorer and richer countries comprise test cases of whether countries can work together to counter shared threats, and a test of the will of those in the World Health Organization (WHO) and elsewhere charged with the global governance and improvement of health.

This high-profile and emotive issue can mask a low-profile and equally difficult issue. As readers of this Journal know better than anyone, the diseases that may in time become great pandemics are more likely to arise and gain a foothold from which to spread to areas and countries that have the least developed health and surveillance systems. There is more chance that they will be undetected for longer, possibly misinterpreted and perhaps, even, deliberately hidden. Moreover, there is a greater chance in such relatively weaker and less regulated health systems that our defenses against such diseases will be compromised, with uncontrolled use of drugs allowing multidrug-resistant strains to arise.

In these circumstances we all have an interest in supporting and strengthening the health systems of our neighbors. Our own self interest, let alone any moral sense or feeling of natural justice, means that we can no longer ignore the health problems of the most disadvantaged areas of the world. Issues that might previously have been seen as part of the substance and subject matter of International Health, and worthy subjects for charity and aid, have become real Global Health concerns for us all.

Our interdependence goes far beyond this. Professor Julio Frenk, the former Minister of Health for Mexico and now Dean of the Harvard School of Public Health, has identified 7 different types of interdependence, all of which need to shape our understanding of Global Health and our response to our shared problems.[2] Here it is worth drawing out 4 categories that go beyond infectious diseases. The first group are the environmental aspects of climate change, pollution, the loss of natural resources and habitats, and overpopulation, which affect us directly in many ways and can, in turn, lead to mass migration, conflict, and disease. The second is the growing incidence of noncommunicable disease, which is increasing in many countries alongside rising wealth and the accompanying change in lifestyles—itself fed by a more global culture that influences our habits—as part of an "epidemiologic transition." The third is the way in which resources which are costly and in short supply—whether they are trained health workers, equipment, or drugs—are distributed, unequally, around the world.

Sitting alongside these 3 is a fourth category, which has received less attention as yet. It concerns our scientific and medical knowledge and the way in which the traditions of Western Scientific Medicine have been, and are being, shaped and spread around the world by the interests of commerce and academia. The important point here is not criticism, far less repudiation, of science and scientific medicine.

Scientific skepticism and objectivity, vide Flexner, is part of the bedrock of health care and health improvement. There is room for a critique, however, of the *way* particular models of health care systems and academic knowledge and teaching are becoming received wisdom around the world. The ways in which science and professional education have developed in Europe and North America are not necessarily the only valid ways. They require challenge. There are different possibilities and traditions and importantly, as argued here, new traditions are being developed. We have a shared interest in how knowledge is developed, managed, and propagated.

Within our medical ecology as much as in the physical environment, we need to understand that diversity offers us some security and that "monocultures" of knowledge as well as of agricultural practice leave us vulnerable.

I will return to this topic at the end of this article, but first wish to explore our interdependence in the context of human resources and discuss how the capacity of the health workforce can be built up globally. Like other resources, trained health workers are not distributed evenly or equitably around the world. **Fig. 1** contrasts the burden of disease and the availability of resources to tackle it between the richest and poorest continents. Sub-Saharan Africa, with slightly more than 10% of the world's population, has 25% of the burden of disease; 3% of the world's health resources and around 1% of the world's trained health workers deal with this burden. North America, with around 5% of the world's population, has about 3% of the burden of disease, 25% of the world's health resources, and 30% of the world's health workers (see **Fig. 1**).

THE HEALTH WORKFORCE

There undoubtedly are important gaps in surveillance in the richest and most developed health systems and countries in the world which need to be addressed; however, they are nothing like as severe or as damaging as the gaps in low-income and middle-income countries. It is important for the safety of us all that health and surveillance systems are strong everywhere. We all have our parts to play.

There is a well-documented shortage of trained health workers globally, with the poorest countries having the greatest shortfalls. The World Health Report for 2006

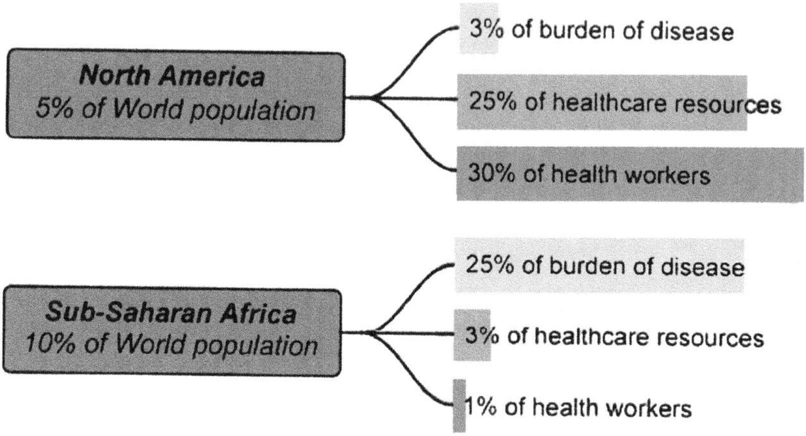

Fig. 1. Comparisons of resources and burdens in the richest and poorest continents. (*From* Crisp N. Turning the world upside down—the search for global health in the 21st century. (London): RSM Press; 2010. p. 30; with permission.)

estimated that there was a global shortfall of at least 4.3 million health workers, and that 57 countries had a critical shortfall.[3]

First, let us look at the composition of the health workforce in these countries. It is immediately apparent that this is very different from the norm in Europe and the United States. Almost throughout the world, from Pakistan with its Lady Health Workers, Brazil with its rural primary care teams, and Ethiopia with its Health Extension Workers, there has been a large increase in the training and deployment of community health workers. These health workers, based in villages and neighborhoods, are able to deal with health at the most local level in ways that cross the boundaries between clinical care and public health. These workers have different responsibilities in different locations but may typically be concerned with clean water, sanitation, immunization, prenatal care, and the treatment of common conditions with a small range of drugs.

Research has shown that these workers can be effective where they are focused on a few roles or tasks, receive good initial training, undergo some level of supervision and follow-up training, and have the knowledge and ability to refer on to higher trained health workers where necessary.[4,5] Part of their strength is that they are in and of the community, and able to link into a variety of informal community structures as well as the more formal facilities and institutions of the local health services. These community health workers provide the first line of defense against—or, if you prefer, attack on—disease, and have the potential to provide some of the information needed in properly surveying the incidence and spread of disease as well as contributing to its containment and control.

In all too many countries, poverty and everything that is associated with it complicates the situation and leads to poor health, and means that completely inadequate health systems are left to face up to today's diseases and to tomorrow's potential pandemics. Health and health care are not stand-alone concepts. Education, housing, and employment are linked to health while strong and vibrant communities are far more resilient in dealing with health and other problems. We know that poor education, high birth rates, unemployment, and social ills such as crime and conflict can contribute to a downward spiral of ill health while improved education (particularly for girls), lower birth rates, safer societies, better nutrition, and growing income can all lead to an upward spiral. Context and community are part of the problem and the solution (**Fig. 2**).

In many countries these community health workers are supported by "mid-level workers," health workers who have been trained in a specific set of tasks or skills

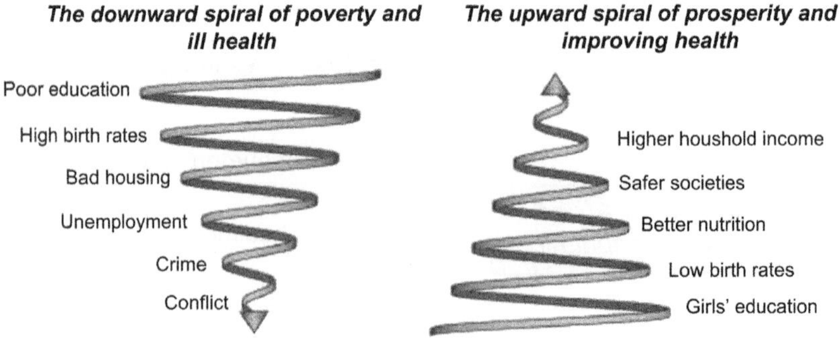

Fig. 2. An illustration of the relationship between poverty and health. (*From* Crisp N. Turning the world upside down—the search for global health in the 21st century. (London): RSM Press; 2010. p. 28; with permission.)

important to a country without receiving a full and lengthy professional training. These workers are given a variety of different titles in different countries including clinical officers, *tecnicos di cirurgia*, and medical officers, and carry out a range of tasks depending on location and priorities, including cesarean sections, trauma, and cataract surgery. They in turn are able to operate most effectively where they have good training and supervision, and are linked in to other more highly trained health professionals. Here again, there is good evidence of how mid-level workers can perform specified tasks to a very high level of competence with, for example, *tecnicos di cirurgia* in Mozambique performing cesarean sections consistently over several years with as few complications as physicians and at lower cost.[6]

The crucial point here is that to be truly effective, community health workers and mid-level workers need to be an integral part of a system sharing in its knowledge, training, protocols, referral pathways, and communications. This ideal position is not realized in many areas and many countries where for reasons ranging from political instability, outright conflict, and widespread poverty, there may be fragmented systems or even none at all. In these circumstances a variety of different project-based and ad hoc approaches may be necessary with teams from government, nongovernmental organizations, and development partners all attempting to fill the gaps.

In the longer term, however, the aim must be to build a broadly based community infrastructure connected to both the informal and formal support systems in the community. This linkage will provide the platform for surveillance and disease management in populations as well as better health care for individuals.

The Global Health Workforce Alliance was set up in 2006 as a response to the World Health Report of that year by the WHO and its partners to advocate for the importance of human resource development, and to identify and spread best practice and the findings of research. It, in turn, created several task forces to review and make recommendations in specific areas. In 2007 it established the Task Force on Education and Training, which was charged with identifying how to accelerate massively the education and training of health workers in those countries in crisis.

The Task Force brought together people from different backgrounds and different countries, and was chaired by the Honourable Bience Gawanas (the African Union Commissioner for Social Affairs) and the author. The Task Force studied successful "scaling-up" processes in 10 countries and produced proposals in its 2008 report *Scaling Up, Saving Lives*[7] on how best to increase the health workforce in all the countries with a critical shortfall. Central to its recommendations was the understanding of the need to produce appropriately trained health workers *and* a functioning health system. The two go hand in hand.

The Task Force concluded that a phased approach was necessary where immediate action could be taken to train more community health workers and reduce attrition from existing training programs. This action would be followed in turn by the longer term training of mid-level workers and the traditional professionals. It would require a good 10 years at least for most countries to become anything like self sufficient in key health workers and to have built up the critical mass of staff and knowledge necessary to support a well-functioning health system. The actual pace at which the workforce could be built up in any country would be determined by the availability of human and financial resources and the supply of employment opportunities for the health workers who had been trained. **Fig. 3** offers an overview of the immediate, mid-term, and longer term actions that might be undertaken as part of such a scaling-up process within a country.

The education and training of more health workers is critical for the successful development of an effective health system, but is not sufficient by itself. Emigration

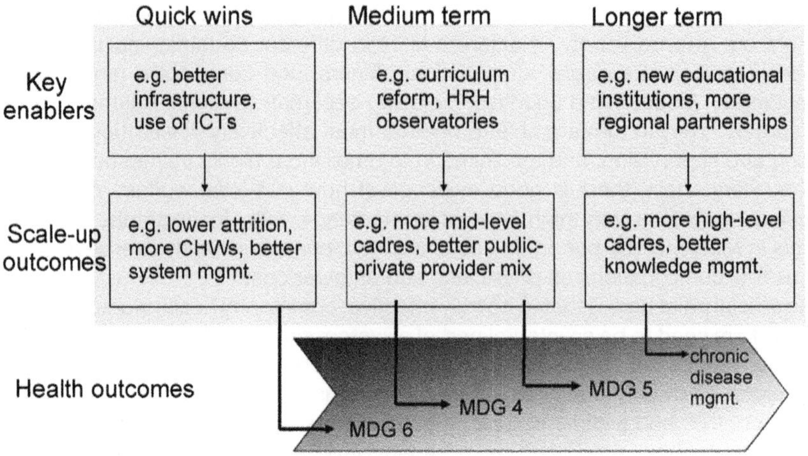

Fig. 3. The 10-year program to build up the health workforce. HRH, Human Resources for Health; MDG, Millennium Development Goals.

of trained health workers from poorer to richer countries, problems of retaining health workers in poorly functioning and badly equipped health facilities, and the lack of money to pay wages all contribute to the difficulties.

At this point it is worth making a temporary excursion into the topic of migration. Migration has been a very damaging phenomenon for many low-income and middle-income countries where a large proportion of recent graduates from nursing and medical schools have left their homelands. At the individual level it is not a simple picture or straightforward story. People have had different motivations to leave. Migration in some cases has been circular—with migrants returning home better equipped to serve the needs of their own countries—and some health workers have moved from one low-income country to another to receive slightly better pay and conditions. The overall picture, however, has been one of movement of trained health workers with their skills and talents moving from poorer environments to richer ones.

The World Health Assembly in May 2010 agreed a Code of Practice[8] for migration, which explicitly recognized both the rights of migrants, who may be denied the right to migrate at home and be exploited abroad, and the responsibilities of countries which were currently benefiting or had in the past benefited extensively from the inward flow of expertise and experience. It proposed, among other things, that these receiving countries should recompense the "exporting" countries by supporting the training of more health workers in these countries.

ROLE OF DEVELOPMENT PARTNERS

This discussion takes us on to the role of development partners in supporting the development of effective health systems in countries that lack them. Part of their role is to advocate for the importance of the development of health systems and provide funding for such development, both within the country—where other priorities may prevail—and within the global community. Another part is, of course, to provide humanitarian assistance where countries are in crisis or in conflict. A further major role is to support the pre-service training and education of health workers to increase the supply.

Migration is an important issue. However, it needs to be seen in proportion. The best estimates suggest that about 135,000 health workers from Sub-Saharan Africa who have received their initial training in their home countries have migrated to richer countries over the last 35 years.[9] This figure is less than 10% of the shortfall of 1.5 million estimated by the WHO to be needed for the Continent. In numerical terms the biggest problem is that not enough health workers are being trained in the first place.

Several high-income countries such as the United Kingdom, the United States, and France, which have benefited from migrant health workers, have excellent traditions of education and training. This is clearly a very significant area where they can and should help by offering assistance to train more health workers in their own countries. This training is happening, but still only in a very patchy and small-scale way.

These development partners also have a role in developing the research, ideas, and technologies that will strengthen health and surveillance systems in countries with few resources of their own. A great deal of international effort is devoted to this from individual governments, international bodies, and philanthropic organizations. While there has been criticism of the slowness of response—and sometimes the lack of fulfillment of promises by donors—we have nevertheless seen the development in recent years of many programs to fund technologies, drugs, and vaccines to address the problems of the poor as opposed to the rich countries and peoples. This social solidarity has benefits for both parties.

TURNING THE WORLD UPSIDE DOWN

Innovation and the development of new ideas is not the sole prerogative of high-income countries. Indeed, as explored by the author in *Turning the World Upside Down*,[1] new ideas and approaches coming from low-income and middle-income countries have the potential to deal with some of the most pressing problems arising in high-income countries. Without the resources and the baggage of tradition and vested interests in rich countries, some people in low-income and middle-income countries are innovating and developing new practices.

There are specific innovations with new low-cost equipment and technologies, and it is no surprise that many of the standard practices in human immunodeficiency virus/AIDS have been developed for and in poorer countries which have suffered most from the condition. Perhaps more importantly, there are general approaches that have been developed, some of which have already been mentioned.

Public health and clinical medicine are brought much closer together. There is far more engagement of the community and of women. Health is not treated as a totally separate issue from education and the ability to earn an income, but rather is considered as part of a person's ability to function as an independent human being. Many services are delivered by social enterprises that belong neither to the public nor private sector. Most challenging of all, mid-level workers who are trained for specific tasks can, under the right circumstances, perform them as safely and effectively, and less expensively, than multicompetent health professionals.

In high-income countries we are challenged by how to provide effective health promotion, by how to link health and social care, by how to deal with the impacts of poverty and disadvantage on health, and by growing costs. It would no more be appropriate to transfer practices directly and without modification from low-income to high-income countries than the other way round, but we can undoubtedly each learn from the other's experiences in developing our own new approaches to meet our current challenges.

There is scope for two-way learning and codevelopment, rather than the one-way transfer of knowledge implied in much of the practice and thinking about international development.

THE FUTURE

These ideas about interdependence and codevelopment are beginning to become more widespread. Many young professionals and students are interested in global health and recognize this interdependence.

These people need to become part of the future education of health professionals, and have already influenced the thinking of the independent Commission on the Education of Health Professionals, which reported in November 2010.[10]

Interdependence, mutuality of learning, codevelopment, new ideas about service delivery, and professional education are ushering in a new way of looking at the world of Health.

SUMMARY

This article explores the idea of global health and the way in which the whole world is increasingly interdependent in terms of health. It argues that high-income countries need to help redress the balance of power and resources around the world, for self interest and self preservation if for no other reason. These countries have a particular responsibility to help support the training of more health workers and to strengthen health systems in low-income and middle-income countries. The article also argues that in this interdependent world, high-income countries can learn a great deal from poorer ones as well as vice versa, and that concepts of mutuality and codevelopment will become increasingly important.

ACKNOWLEDGMENTS

I am indebted to my researcher, Susana Edjang, for her support with the research for this article, to many audiences over the last year who have engaged me in debate about these ideas and, above all, to my wife Sian for her unfailing support.

REFERENCES

1. Crisp N. Turning the world upside down—the search for global health in the 21st century. (London): RSM Press; 2010. p. 105.
2. Frenk J, Gomez-Dantes O, Chacon F. Global health in transition, . Handbook of global public health. (London): Routledge; 2010.
3. World Health Organisation. Working together for better health. World Health Organisation (WHO); May 2006.
4. Haines A, Sanders D, Lehman U, et al. Achieving child survival goals: potential contribution of community health workers. Lancet 2007;369(9579):2121–31.
5. Douthewaite M, Ward P. Increasing contraceptive use in rural Pakistan: an evaluation of the Lady Health worker Programme. Health Policy Plan 2005;20(2): 117–23.
6. Pereira A, Cumbi C, Malalane R, et al. Meeting the need for emergency obstetric care in Mozambique: work performance and history of medical doctors and assistant medical officers trained for surgery. Br J Obstet Gynaecol 1997;114: 1253–60.
7. Global Health Workforce Alliance. Scaling up, saving lives. Global Health Workforce Alliance (GHWA); May 2008.

8. World Health Organisation. The WHO Global Code of Practice on the International Recruitment of Health Personnel. World Health Organisation. May, 2010.
9. International Labour Office. Report of the Committee of Migrant Workers, Provisional Record 22, 92nd Session. International Labour Conference, Geneva (Switzerland), June 15–17, 2004.
10. Frenk J, Chen L, Bhutta ZA, et al. Health professionals for a new century: transforming education to strengthen health systems in an interdependent world. Lancet 2010;376(9756):1923–58.

The Infectious Diseases Institute at Makerere University, Kampala, Uganda

Allan Ronald, MD, FRCPC[a,b,*], Moses Kamya, MBBS, MMed, MSc, PhD[b], Elly Katabira, MBBS, MMed, FRCP(Edin)[b], W. Michael Scheld, MD[b,c], Nelson Sewankambo, MBBS, MMed[b]

KEYWORDS

• Uganda • HIV/AIDS training • Leadership development
• Knowledge translation • HIV/AIDS cohorts

THE ORIGIN OF THE INFECTIOUS DISEASE INSTITUTE

We could begin with the human immunodeficiency virus (HIV) epidemic in Africa or the remarkable Ugandan academic leadership that rebuilt Makerere School of Medicine after the civil wars. However, this story begins with Merle Sande. His vision together with that of Makerere School of Medicine Dean, Nelson Sewankambo, and Pfizer Incorporated Pharmaceuticals Chief Executive Officer (CEO), Hank McKinnell, conceived the idea of the Infectious Diseases Institute (IDI) in 2001.

Merle Sande was a uniquely effective leader. Throughout his academic career, he had the capacity to use the power of persuasion to sell ideas. In 2000, throughout the Western world, the care of patients with AIDS had been transformed by antiretroviral treatment (ART). Merle had advocated for access to care for patients with AIDS when he served as Chair of Medicine at San Francisco General Hospital. At the International AIDS Society Conference in South Africa in August 2000, President Nelson Mandela pleaded for the world to respond to the millions dying from AIDS in sub-Saharan Africa. That month Merle summoned 3 colleagues (Jerry Ellner, Tom Quinn, and Allan Ronald) and challenged us to join him as comrades in arms in a shared effort to limit the consequences of the African AIDS epidemic. Subsequently Mike Scheld, another of Merle's confidents, joined the group. Merle and Mike as members of

[a] Department of Medicine, University of Manitoba, C5124-409 Tache Avenue, Winnipeg, Manitoba R2H 2A6, Canada
[b] Department of Medicine, Makerere University, PO Box 7072, Kampala, Uganda
[c] Department of Medicine, University of Virginia, MR 6, Room 2528-345 Crispell Drive, Charlottesville, VA 22908, USA
* Corresponding author. Department of Medicine, University of Manitoba, C5124-409 Tache Avenue, Winnipeg, Manitoba R2H 2A6, Canada.
E-mail address: aronald@ms.umanitoba.ca

doi:10.1016/j.idc.2011.02.007
id.theclinics.com
0891-5520/11/$ – see front matter

Pfizer's Infectious Disease Advisory Board, convinced the leaders at Pfizer Inc of the need for infrastructure and training to address HIV/AIDS in Africa.

In 2000 it seemed futile. The annual cost of ART in North America was in excess of $10,000; logistical systems were not in place to move diagnostics and drugs from manufacturers to patients; AIDS was among the most complex infections managed by infectious disease clinicians. Individuals from the Pfizer Foundation shared their frustrations surrounding efforts to provide fluconazole freely, for patients with life-threatening fungal infections. South Africa had refused to accept the drug, presumably because of a lack of trust of a multinational pharmaceutical company.

However, Merle, Mike, and Hank McKinnell, the incoming CEO of Pfizer Inc, had long-standing friendships. Hank agreed to support our effort and expressed his commitment stating "If we're not part of the solution, we're part of the problem." Discussions commenced with Dean Sewankambo at Makerere School of Medicine. In June 2001, 14 academic colleagues (9 from Uganda, 4 from the United States, and 1 from Canada) met in Kampala. The group agreed on an academic public/private partnership in which the Makerere Medical School, the Mulago Teaching Hospital, the Ministry of Health, and Pfizer Inc with the Pfizer Foundation would work together to establish an IDI at Makerere University. President Yoweri Museveni joined the group and promised his support. The founders named themselves the Academic Alliance for AIDS Care and Prevention in Africa (AA) and are listed in **Box 1**. The AA agreed that a collaborative African-based and African-led initiative to build health care infrastructure and capacity was essential to address the HIV epidemic in sub-Saharan Africa. However, although our primary focus was HIV, from the outset the intention was to address the entire spectrum of infectious diseases that were contributing to the poverty, illness, and early death for so many in sub-Saharan Africa. Breaking the cycle required a collaborative sustained partnership using the principles and

Box 1
Founding members of the academic alliance

North America

- Gerrold Ellner
- Thomas Quinn
- Allan Ronald
- Merle Sande
- Michael Scheld

Uganda

- Nelson Sewankambo
- Moses Kamya
- Elly Katabira
- Edward Katongole-Mbidde
- Harriet Mayanja-Kizza
- Rory Mugerwa
- Philippa Musoke
- David Serwadda
- Fred Wabwire-Mangen

expertise of private sector entrepreneurs along with the science and capacity-building energy of academicians.[1]

The HIV epidemic in Uganda has been well documented.[2–5] One of the founders of the AA, David Serwadda, along with Nelson, described in 1985, the appearance in Uganda of slim disease.[2] In January 1986 Musevani and his revolutionary movement ended the civil war. Shortly thereafter he sent 60 of his officers to Cuba for military training. Sixteen were found to be HIV positive, and Cuban President Fidel Castro suggested to President Museveni that he should pay attention to this new devastating disease. As Museveni tells the story, he has made HIV/AIDS a priority at every opportunity, informing Ugandans about the "lion in the village." As a result, in Uganda HIV became a widely recognized illness and AIDS became a mentionable common cause of death. By 1992 the epidemic in Uganda was generalized, presumably fueled by the disruptions of the civil war and the low (less than 20%) male circumcision rate. Prevalence in prenatal sentinel populations varied around the country between 10% and 25%, with an overall prevalence about 20%.[3,4] At that time Uganda had the highest HIV prevalence anywhere and AIDS was devastating society. The AIDS Support Organization (TASO) and the AIDS Information Center were effective Ugandan responses created to support positive clients and identify HIV-infected individuals. Philly Lutaaya, a globally famous Ugandan musician, became ill with AIDS and spent several years informing Ugandans about the disease. The Joint Clinical Research Center (JCRC) had been created in 1991 by President Museveni as a site for AIDS care and research. Its Director, Peter Mugyenyi, was leading these programs. A research site in the Rakai District of Uganda had been established by Nelson Sewankambo, David Serwadda, Fred Wabwire-Mangen, and colleagues from Johns Hopkins University and they had generated much of our current knowledge about HIV epidemiology in Africa. The Ugandan Virology Research Institute and the British Medical Research Council Laboratories, both in Entebbe, were each making significant research contributions. However, all these remarkable organizations were remote from the Makerere University and Mulago Hospital site, where undergraduate and postgraduate education took place.

After our launch in June 2001, Merle and Nelson accepted the coleadership of AA. Principles articulated early in the program are summarized in **Box 2**. Other articles have described the initial years of the AA.[1,6–8]

Merle Sande was seminal to our success. Although he died of multiple myeloma in November 2007, his legacy influences today's decisions. Some of his characteristics were summarized by his colleague, Dr Warner Greene: "Informality with a purpose; a master clinician; a superb partner especially when he was in charge; an educator and mentor to the world; a dreamer who made dreams come true; a man of great passion and intellect; 'no' was never an option." Merle had an ability to create a presence even when he was busy elsewhere and he had the audacity to take on the impossible. He was also effective at focused delegation with regular accountability. Merle and Nelson began the weekly AA Thursday morning teleconferences, which continue to the present, enabling the AA to be updated and involved. Merle made 4 or 5 trips to Uganda annually, traveling economy class and living out of a suitcase for 2 to 3 months each year, while chairing the Department of Medicine at Utah. He also directed that $1 million of his estate be combined with an equivalent gift from Hank McKinnell to provide a $2 million endowment for the salary of the Executive Director of IDI.

The other leaders who created IDI, Nelson Sewankambo and Hank McKinnell, are equally remarkable. Nelson after graduation from Makerere in 1976 completed training in internal medicine and remained in Uganda through the civil wars. He became Dean in 1990 and provided stellar leadership as the Faculty reorganized and emerged from

Box 2
The principles of the AA

- We endeavor to pursue excellence in science, education, and clinical care within the limited resources available to a society.
- We pursue our goals within the established academic and Ministry of Health structures to enhance and facilitate their goals.
- Our primary responsibility is to enable Africans to achieve their potential as physicians, scientists, educators, and/or administrators and to be mentored as they mature into effective leaders within Africa.
- We recognize the inherent human quality of all individuals and that patients must be treated with dignity, respect, and sensitivity.
- We value bidirectional training with health care providers from both African and Western countries being provided with the opportunity to learn how to improve health in Africa.
- We respect the contributions of both Africans and expatriates but recognize that our primary responsibility is to African trainees.
- We believe that health care must be based on evidence and wherever possible, this evidence needs to be acquired within the appropriate context in Africa.
- We are committed to a sound, fair, transparent, fiscal infrastructure.

the years of repression. He has received numerous accolades including an Honorary Degree of Laws from McMaster University. He currently serves as Principal of the Makerere College of Health Sciences.

Dr Hank McKinnell graduated from Stanford with a PhD in Business. His career at Pfizer culminated with his recruitment in 2001 to the position of CEO. He was an effective advocate within Pfizer for expanding its global health footprint with innovative programs. However, Dr McKinnell and Pfizer gave more than money. In particular, Hank was committed to leadership development. He also had a passion for HIV prevention and reminded us that unless prevention is our overarching priority, the demands of care could not be sustained. Dr McKinnell, with his partner Joanna, made annual trips to Africa, influenced his friends in both the corporate and personal world to support IDI, and accepted the Chair of the Academic Alliance Foundation.

BUILDING IDI AND ITS PROGRAMS

With secure funding and the signing of formal agreements, program development and planning for a building commenced. The Pangaea Global AIDS Foundation in San Francisco was selected by Pfizer and the AA to disburse and be accountable for funds donated by Pfizer. Barbara Lawton, the Pangaea program director, ensured that schedules were followed. A Canadian couple, Charles Wilson and Julia Martin, were recruited to be responsible, with African colleagues, for constructing the building and developing programs. Allan Ronald had recently retired from the University of Manitoba and with his wife Myrna resided in Uganda for 3 years and assisted in program development.

The challenges were daunting and on many occasions failure appeared to be the most probable outcome. Philosophic differences between the Pangaea Foundation and the AA had to be addressed and resolved. Formal agreements for the land and ultimately for the operation of IDI as a semiautonomous organization, with its own grants management, human resource, and finance infrastructure had to be painstakingly developed with clarity and official approval at multiple levels. Charles Wilson had excellent negotiating skills and with Dean Sewankambo established a solid foundation with a mutually acceptable memorandum of understanding. The architectural design of the new facility was planned within the Kampala environment with AA colleagues. It was the first new building on the medical school site in more than 30 years. Construction was completed in 2005. It has proved to be an excellent base for IDI programs, with 15 examining rooms, an excellent reception area, exceptional patient flow logistics, conference rooms that can be modified and coalesced, substantial administrative space, and a well-designed laboratory. Security, electrical back-up systems, well-sited washrooms, and creative flexibility were all important parts of the design. In an average week, approximately 5000 individuals enter the building as patients, students, employees, care providers, researchers, and visitors.

THE CLINICAL PROGRAMS

Professor Elly Katabira had initiated the first HIV clinic in Africa (the Mulago Immunodeficiency Clinic) in 1987. Patients were counseled and received care for opportunistic infections. However, without ART, most patients died of AIDS. Allan Ronald joined this clinic and additional space was obtained, medical officers, nurses, counselors and a dispensing technologist were recruited, and daily clinics begun. By December 2002, more than 2000 patients with HIV were registered. However, fewer than a hundred were on ART and these were usually on self-purchased regimens that were often incongruous and frequently depended on supplies sent by the Ugandan diaspora. Visitors from the West had to learn that active tuberculosis (TB) was present in most of the patients with advanced HIV; patients presented with cryptococcal meningitis almost daily; Kaposi sarcoma was highly prevalent; and the usual bacterial infections seen in North America were common. Shared learning experiences were created. Case presentations and the research hour became part of the weekly schedule. Limited ART became available with the Multi-Country Access Program of the World Bank in June 2004 and in 2005 900 slots of free ART became available through the President's Emergency Plan for AIDS Relief.

Once the program moved to the IDI building in 2005, the numbers on care expanded exponentially. This development was in part because of the initiation of routine testing in Mulago Hospital that led to the identification of large numbers of HIV-infected individuals.[9] It became obvious that the number of patients who needed care and treatment at Mulago Hospital could not possibly be met by IDI. Our capacity was overwhelmed and our training and research mandates could be compromised. In 2006 IDI implemented innovative strategies to handle the increasing volumes of patients. These strategies can be summarized as follows:

- Internal efforts to increase clinic efficiency through task shifting. As the patients' quality of life improved on medications, categories of clinic visits that do not require a doctor were introduced in a systematic criteria-driven way by Charles Steinberg, one of the US trainers. This strategy enabled the doctors to attend to more complicated cases and reduced transit time of patients through the clinic.
- External initiative, through the development of a referral system with Kampala City Council (KCC) health facilities, HIV care capacity was built and patients were transferred to these facilities.

Currently more than 10,000 active people living with HIV/AIDS (PHAs) are followed up at the IDI clinic, with 7000 on ART. Almost half of the clinic visits at IDI are nurse visits and pharmacy refill visits. Furthermore, an additional 7300 PHAs are receiving care from the 6 KCC regional clinics that IDI has supported and 2900 are on ART. These strategies have enabled IDI to provide HIV care services to more than 17,000 PHAs, or about 5% of the national HIV care burden.

To improve care at IDI, additional services were added, including a clinic for integrated management of TB, a Kaposi sarcoma clinic, and family planning services. A dedicated clinic for young adults was also established to meet the needs of adolescents as they made the transition to adulthood and services to support discordant couples were launched to promote HIV prevention.

The clinic has been the venue for more than 50 research studies. Hundreds of undergraduate and postgraduate students at Makerere University as well as students, residents, and fellows from Western institutions have had clinical rotations and mentorship within the clinic.

In 2004 Bob Colebunders from The Institute of Tropical Medicine at the University of Antwerp took a year's sabbatical with IDI. He made substantial contributions to training particularly through facilitating individuals to acquire postgraduate degrees in Antwerp while continuing their research in Uganda. He has continued to be a major contributor to the programs. Ceppie Merry, a pharmacokinetics scientist from Dublin, came to initiate studies on antiretrovirals and stayed to be our resident drug expert. Walter Schlech from Dalhousie University and Paul Bohjanen from Minnesota in University of Minnesota came as trainers and returned on multiple occasions as researchers and professors-in-residence.

Initially IDI included pediatrics in its program. By 2004 more than 100 adolescent HIV-infected patients had registered for care. Most of these were long-term survivors of HIV acquired at birth or in infancy. Most were orphans and struggling with declining health, few opportunities to secure an education, and limited, if any, family support. Marshalling resources for these teens and obtaining ART became a priority. Since 2006 Baylor University, with financial support from Bristol Meyers Squibb, has taken responsibility for the pediatric and adolescent programs.

Laboratory services are essential for the care of seriously ill patients with infections. Too often these services are not readily available.[10] The Johns Hopkins Department of Pathology had established a research laboratory in 1991 within the Mulago Hospital complex. This laboratory moved into IDI in 2005 and serves research, patient care, and training needs under the managerial leadership of Ali Elbirer. In 2010, 78 research protocols were under way and more than 160,000 tests performed. In addition, Dr Moses Joloba, Chair of Makerere's Department of Microbiology has developed, with the support of Becton Dickinson and IDI, a laboratory training course for African laboratory managers and bench technologists.

Infectious disease fellowships are not available for medical graduates in sub-Saharan African.[11] In a learning environment in which most admissions to medical and pediatric wards are ill with infections, African physicians are expected to manage these well. However, without infectious disease academic faculty, clinical microbiology is not adequately valued and there is little excitement around infectious disease issues.[10,11] One of our initial goals was to develop and mentor trainees in this discipline. Andrew Kambugu and David Meya (**Fig. 1**) were the initial 2 trainees and both have performed exceptionally well as young clinician scientists. They have recently received their initial RO1 from the US National Institutes of Health (NIH) for studies on cryptococcal meningitis. Many more infectious diseases graduates are required to provide care for complicated infections including advanced HIV, liaise and support Ministry of Health Public Health programs, and carry out the academic mission.

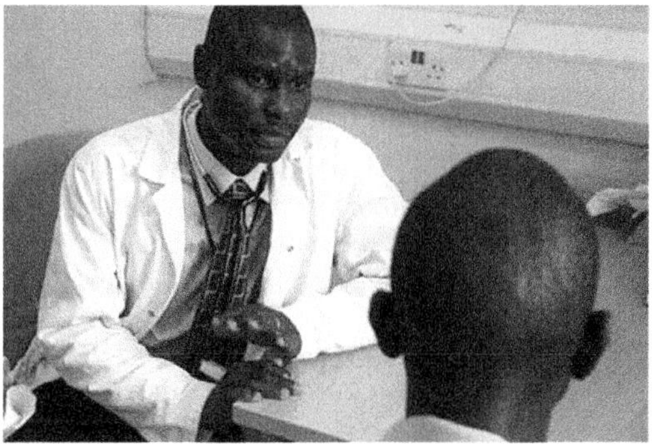

Fig. 1. Dr David Meya is a Makerere graduate who completed his medical residency in internal medicine with his master's degree and embarked on a 3-year infectious disease fellowship at IDI and at the University of Minnesota. During that time he acquired skills in molecular biology, specifically microarray gene technology. He also, with colleagues from Minnesota and Dr Andrew Kambugu, developed initiatives in cryptococcal disease management. These initiatives are already improving the care of this disease within Uganda. He is a busy scientist with an NIH grant. With his responsibilities on the Mulago medical wards and at IDI, his days are full. However, he does continue to find time to spend with his physician wife and their 3 children. IDI and Accordia hope that David will be joined by many other infectious disease physicians over the next decade. "Accordia and IDI are making tremendous strides in changing the way we address the challenges of infectious diseases in Africa. IDI is a place where young African scientists can learn how to confront infectious disease epidemics in our setting."

HIV/AIDS TRAINING

Our initial mission was "to build capacity for delivering sustainable quality HIV/AIDS care and prevention for Africa through training and research." Shortly after our launch, a curriculum appropriate for primary care providers was crafted. Trainers are recruited through the ranks of the Infectious Diseases Society of America (IDSA) and applications are available on the IDSA Web site.

From their inception, all training programs include pretests and posttests as well as obligations of each trainee to research a topic comprehensively. In addition to the lectures, the training also includes telemedicine presentations, small group discussions, seminars, case studies, journal club discussions, interactive sessions, and active Web-based learning with real cases through Internet access. Each trainee receives a course binder that includes all slides from the lectures delivered and copies of journal articles discussed. Over time, didactic instruction has been dramatically reduced. The training includes clinical placements at Mulago adult and pediatric wards, the JCRC, Mildmay International, and other sites in Kampala. The first class, consisting of 12 trainees, was enrolled in April 2002 and was expanded to 25 in 2004. Gisela Schneider, a German missionary with extensive experience in African health care, was recruited in 2005 to expand training programs to other infectious diseases and to include nurses, clinical officers, laboratory technologists, and other health professionals.

The Joint Uganda Malaria Program was launched in 2007 with funding from Exxon Mobile and the leadership of Moses Kamya and colleagues from the University of California San Francisco. This 1-week course focuses on malaria exclusively and introduced "cluster training, allowing medical officers, nurses and laboratory technologists from the same facility to train together in the prevention and management of malaria.

Rigorous preevaluation and postevaluation of malaria care showed a dramatic increase in diagnosis and appropriate management.

In 2009 the integrated management of infectious diseases training course began. This is the core training component of the Infectious Disease Capacity (IDCAP) building program codirected by Lydia Mpanga Sebuyrira, Marcia Weaver, Sarah Naikoba, and Kelly Willis. IDCAP is funded by the Bill and Melinda Gates Foundation (BMGF) and designed to determine the most cost-effective method for training midlevel practitioners (clinical officers and nurses) in sub-Saharan Africa. These cadres deliver most clinical care in this region. It is administered by the Accordia Global Health Foundation in cooperation with IDI, the Makerere University College of Health Sciences, the International Training and Education Center on HIV at the University of Washington, and the Uganda Ministry of Health. A Curriculum Committee, chaired by Ian Crozier, created the 3-week case-based curriculum. Although HIV/AIDS, malaria, and TB constitute most of the curriculum, all common infectious diseases in Uganda are included. IDCAP also is evaluating on-site support via a 5-member mobile team who visit the IDCAP sites. A clinical decision guide consisting of algorithms for management of the most common infectious diseases encountered in sub-Saharan Africa is provided to each trainee. The AA has also ensured that lessons learned from our educational efforts are peer-reviewed.[12]

From the humble beginning of 12 students enrolled in the first class in April 2002, the IDI Training Program has now trained more than 6000 African health care workers from 27 African countries. The Training Program is now under the leadership of Dr Lydia Mpanga Sebuyrira, who directs a staff of 14.

THE ACCORDIA FOUNDATION AND THE EVOLUTION OF THE AA

Merle Sande, with support from Hank McKinnell and Pfizer Inc, created the Academic Alliance Foundation in 2003. It was renamed Accordia Global Foundation in 2008. Accordia serves as the institutional home of AA and has overseen the growth and development of IDI as a center of excellence. Initially, this included recruiting senior management, developing programs, establishing governance structures, liaising with corporate partners, and fund-raising. Individuals with global health expertise, business acumen, and a passion for Africa were identified to serve on the Board. In 2007, Merle and Hank requested their colleague, Dr Warner Greene, Director of the Gladstone Center for Virology and Immunology and the Nick and Sue Hellmon Distinguished Professor of Translational Medicine at the University of California at San Francisco, to assume leadership of the Foundation. Since 2007 Carol Spahn has been the Executive Director.

Over the past 3 years Accordia's role has shifted as IDI has become increasingly self-sufficient. Accordia is now leading targeted research activities and has been tasked with increasing responsibility for partnering with other nongovernmental organizations, universities, and the private sector, advocating for health resources for Africa, and assisting with IDI program expansion. Its mandate includes the development of other African-owned and African-led centers of excellence. The AA group continues to meet by teleconference weekly, supports IDI in multiple ways, and attends the annual review sessions. New Ugandan, American, and European academicians have been recruited to the group, now with 21 individuals sharing responsibility under the leadership of the AA cochairs, Nelson Sewankambo and Michael Scheld. Many of the AA members spend 2 to 4 weeks each year as professors-in-residence. This program combines teaching rounds at Mulago Hospital with attending in IDI, participating in clinical and research activities, and mentoring young Ugandans.

Establishing a Research Program

Research at IDI is conducted by teams of investigators, funded by external research agencies, and bolstered by state-of-the-art data management capabilities and a College of American Pathology-certified laboratory.

In 2002 the AA obtained a BMGF grant to begin a research program. Led by Professors Fred Wabwire-Mangen, Elly Katabira, and Allan Ronald (principal investigators), a series of clinic and population-based initiatives to inform patient care and strengthen HIV prevention was performed. Studies in the HIV clinic investigated headache, visual problems, hepatic disease, cryptococcal disease, dementia, and adolescent HIV.[13–17] New HIV prevention messages and materials were developed and produced. An AIDS Treatment and Information Center was established to provide a distance electronic forum for discussion on HIV care. Other research funded by this grant included studies on adherence to antiretrovirals, the testing of innovative laboratory techniques to support laboratory monitoring of HIV treatment in resource-limited settings, and an HIV behavioral surveillance trend analysis.[18–20] However, the major outcome of this grant was the creation of the research infrastructure at IDI (**Fig. 2**). A cadre of medical officers and nurses acquired skill in research processes. Colleagues from the West became coinvestigators on subsequent grants to NIH and European granting bodies. Thirty peer-reviewed manuscripts have arisen from this initial BMGF funding.

In 2003 IDI joined the DART (Development of Antiretroviral Therapy in Africa) Trial, a multisite study led by Dr Peter Mugyenyi designed to give insights into HIV monitoring strategies in resource-limited settings. The trial randomized 3300 patients with AIDS to routine versus only clinically driven monitoring of antiretroviral therapy.[21]

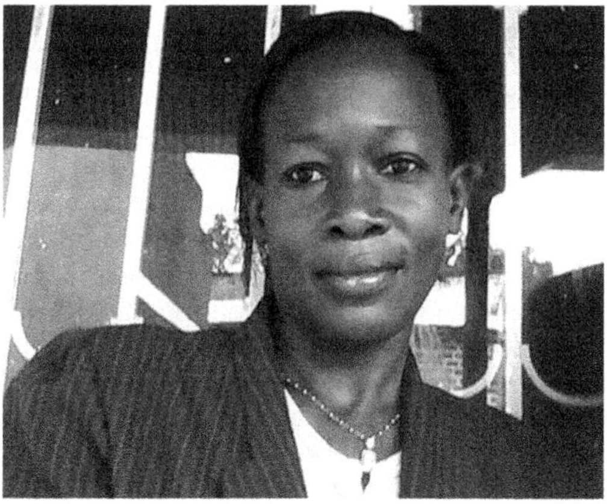

Fig. 2. Alice Namudge is a nurse who was recruited in 2002 initially to work in the clinic and to perform psychoneurologic studies on patients with HIV with cognitive impairment. Alice is HIV positive and has coped with numerous complications of the disease and its treatment. Initially she presented with wasting and diarrhea in 1998. Subsequently she had both cryptococcal meningitis and toxoplasmosis. In 2002 her hemoglobin dropped to 2.2 g on azidothymidine; on d4T she developed severe neuropathy and was wheelchair-bound for 6 months. She was also diagnosed with TB and developed optic atrophy on ethambutol. IDI assumed her care in 2003 and she has returned to normal health with a CD4 count of 870 and is a healthy, happy, active participant in IDI programs. She has been able to purchase land and build a house for her son and herself as well as 2 orphan nephews. She states "IDI has met all my expectations and I am able to encourage other patients because I've been there too."

Neither arm included viral load testing. The DART study enabled 301 patients from IDI, many within months of death, to receive ART when none was otherwise available. Only 4% of the IDI patients were lost to follow up and 234 were alive and most were well 5 years after initiating ART.

In 2004 Moses Kamya assembled a prospective observation cohort of 1000 HIV-infected patients to further understand the effectiveness and outcomes of ART.[22] IDI has focused its efforts on operational research to develop best practice models. Multiple groups have partnered IDI to conduct clinical and epidemiologic studies focused on these databases.[23,24]

David Thomas from Johns Hopkins was recruited in 2005 to be the Director of Research at IDI. He was followed in 2006 by Phillippa Easterbrook from Imperial College and in 2007 by Yuka Manabe from Hopkins. Each contributed with Ugandan partners to the creation of the research infrastructure, enabling ongoing skills enhancement and creating new programs.

Externally funded research under way at IDI in 2010 included studies on TB diagnostics (Moses Joloba, Yuka Manabe, Harriet Mayanja, and Jerry Ellner), TB immune reconstitution, inflammatory syndrome (IRIS) and immunology (Bob Colebunders, Harriet Mayanja, William Worodria, and Yuka Manabe), cryptococcal disease management and IRIS (Andrew Kambugu, David Meya, Paul Bohjanen, David Boulware, and Edward Janoff),[25] genital herpes suppression and pre-exposure prophylaxis in discordant couples (Connie Celum, Jared Baetan, Elly Katabira, Edith Nakku, and Allan Ronald)[26,27] drug pharmacokinetics (Ceppie Merry, Mohammed Lamorde, and Pauline Byakikia-Kibwika),[28] bacterial sepsis management (Mike Scheld, Shevin Jacob, Gyanviira Makanga, and Chris Moore),[29] Kaposi sarcoma (Jeff Martin and Edward Mbidde), human herpesvirus 8 epidemiology (Cory Casper and Jackson Orem),[30] HIV dementia (Ned Sachtor and Noeline Nakasujja)[31] hepatitis B epidemiology and management (Ponsiano Ocama, Kenneth Opio, Stephen Reynolds, and David Thomas), and others. More than 100 manuscripts have now been written and the 2010 research budget approximated 4 million dollars.

Training and capacity building, through the development of promising young investigators, are the cornerstone of this program. The IDI strategy was designed based on a recommendation made by the Uganda National Health Research Organization: to create and strengthen a critical mass of human resources capable of planning and implementing research projects that address national health needs. Through these programs, 16 PhD candidates and more than 20 Masters students are supported by IDI.

The Gilead Sciences Sewankambo Scholar Program was designed in 2007 to be an extension of postdoctoral clinical training. It aims to train new, independent, internationally competitive clinical investigators at Makerere University over an intensive 5-year period. Applicants selected receive full funding for 5 years and devote 70% of their effort to research and career development. Scholars are expected to write at least 5 peer-reviewed papers and to have become a principal investigator. Investigators have access to resources to enable them to conduct research, undertake clinical research training courses, and present their findings at local and international meetings.

An International Scientific Advisory Board was established to advise IDI. It is composed of respected scientists from the United States, Europe, and Africa and was chaired initially by King Holmes and currently by Paul Volberding. In addition, AA members mentor and shape research capacity-building programs.

IDI has built a vibrant research capacity. More than 600 individuals have taken research and statistics courses within IDI. Together we foster an environment where critical appraisal occurs in a collaborative, comfortable, and collegial environment.

More importantly, IDI is developing the next generation of Ugandan leaders in health science.

The McAdam Era (2004–2007)

In 2004 Professor Keith McAdam was recruited to be the initial Executive Director of IDI. He had previously been Professor of Clinical Tropical Medical at the London School of Hygiene and Tropical Medicine and Director of the Medical Research Laboratory in the Gambia. Keith, with Nelson's support, carefully set in place the structures that have governed and sustained IDI to date. He established an independent IDI Board and recruited a Senior Management Team, after international searches. This team included Directors of Administration, Development, Training, Research, Clinical Services, the Laboratory and Information Services. Keith also set in place clearly defined expectations for all senior staff members. He ensured that there were internal and external audits, continuing development of skills in managing both human and fiscal resources, and standard operating practices. Keith also had a profound effect on the clinics at IDI through his personal involvement. Patients became "our friends" (*mikwano gyaffe* in Luganda) and numerous programs were developed to facilitate peer support as well as opportunity for learning entrepreneurial and life skills. These programs enabled "our friends" to gain hope, confidence, and self-employment and shed the stigma of HIV.

During these 3 years, research support grew rapidly and as noted earlier, the clinical load increased dramatically. Keith obtained the initial large development grant for IDI to transform the Kampala City Health Clinics through training and support activities. This strategy also enabled IDI to transfer care for "our friends" to clinics nearer their residences and reduce the burgeoning IDI patient load.

The Coutinho Years (Since 2007)

Alex Coutinho succeeded Keith McAdam as the Executive Director of IDI in 2007. He graduated from Makerere University Medical School, obtained graduate training in Emergency Medicine, Health Service Management, and Public Health at the University of Witwatersrand and then developed and administrated health programs in Swaziland. In 2001 he was recruited to lead TASO, which by 2007 provided resources to more than 100,000 HIV-infected individuals throughout Uganda. Since its creation in 1987 by Noerine Kaleeba TASO has enabled PHAs to take charge of their lives, access prevention and care programs, and escape poverty.[32] During his initial 3 years at IDI, Alex has built on the foundation established by Merle, Nelson, Hank, Keith, and others and rapidly expanded programs. In particular, his relationships with the Ministry of Health, the academic community, and the donor community have enabled him to secure program contracts. The Kiboga/Kibale program is 1 such example. These 2 districts in Western Uganda are large agricultural areas with limited health facilities. More than 40% of the health staff positions were unfilled. Within the first 18 months 188,000 individuals were counseled and tested for HIV, 8000 individuals were provided with HIV care, and 2400 individuals started on ART. Alex relates effectively to individuals and organizations and has been able to raise philanthropic as well as donor monies. Space is an acute problem, with administrative and research space spread over 5 different sites. As a result, he has led a planning initiative to build a new facility on the Makerere University campus. This new 9-storey building with an attached auditorium will enable all IDI administrative and training activities to be housed in 1 facility. It will be convenient to the existing IDI site at Mulago Hospital, which will continue to provide patient care and conduct clinical research. The new facility will cost about $6 million and fund-raising is under way.

Dr Coutinho has also directed IDI activities into the mainstream of Makerere University College of Health Sciences and the Ministry of Health, including Mulago Hospital. IDI has supported Mulago in improving health care through support to infrastructure renovations, equipment, and staff time to consult on the medical wards. Our success depends on a strategy to continually enhance the effectiveness and efficiency of both these organizations, which have the major responsibilities to lead health professional education and health care programs. Also, Dr Coutinho has established a strong link with Gulu University and provided educational resources.

The Contribution of IDI to Makerere University and its College of Health Sciences

Since 1995 Makerere University has been rebuilding itself after the brutal years of dictatorship. IDI has contributed to regaining Makerere Medical School's previous status as a national asset with an international reputation where people interact in the quest for excellent science and health professional education.

IDI is a crucible for experimentation in management systems within the health academic environment and it opened a new era of decentralization in university governance and management. IDI was given authority to function as a limited company within the University with its own human resource policies and freedom to hire local and expatriate personnel on its own terms and conditions. It was also allowed to raise the needed financial resources. This experiment has enhanced the spirit of innovations at the College and the University as a whole.

Today the College of Health Sciences with the backing and support from the University is developing its institutional management. The partnership that has been nurtured between academia and the private sector at IDI has brought to the fore the importance of these collaborations. The University and the College are both increasingly receptive to new ideas because of the success of the IDI model.

IDI has also added 780 square meters (8400 square feet) of critically needed space. The laboratory at IDI has also won international awards in recognition of its high performance standards, a clear illustration that excellence can be achieved.

The overall outputs of the College are enhanced because of the benefits accruing from academic and administrative infrastructure available at IDI. The College and IDI are becoming known for their attention to issues of social accountability and fulfilling their social mission as an academic center.[33] With its information technology infrastructure supported by NIH, the College has been able to use videoconferencing and benefit the Makerere community through seminars between our students and faculty in other universities.

The AA, IDI, and Accordia Foundation as Change Agents

What unique strategies other than a grand vision, industrious individuals, and substantial resources have made the initial 10 years a success? All 3 organizations have been opportunistic and pragmatic, facilitating change and adhering to their initial principles. Hybrid leaders have been created who represent some of the best elements of African and Western academic cultures. We have listened to and respected each other. We have worked from within Makerere University and Mulago Hospital to strengthen and enable the success of their educational and care structures and we have worked closely with the Ministry of Health to facilitate its mission. Although the creation of new science and the use of evidence in health policies and practice is our primary characteristic, our major transformative success story has been the identification and support of capable young leaders who are assuming roles at IDI as well as within academic positions elsewhere. They are the future and will ensure that the infectious diseases burden is reduced in Africa.

The Second Decade

Our consortium has worked collaboratively to achieve our primary goals at IDI to:

- promote sustainable cost-effective, high-quality infectious disease prevention and care with an emphasis on HIV/AIDS
- pursue biomedical research and build research capacity to further the understanding and knowledge of infectious disease in Africa
- translate medical advances by training African clinicians and public health providers to markedly reduce infectious disease consequences in Africa.

These goals continue to be our priority. However, our vision now incorporates a broader framework to partner other countries in Africa. Our emphasis includes medical education, building academic capacity (including infrastructure and leadership), and focusing on big picture problems (particularly implementing and scaling up HIV prevention). Collaboration between African institutions is facilitated. Mentorship and an ongoing critical evaluation of all programs to ensure an excellent return on the investment remain at the core of all of these activities. An expanding vision into the broader African context will lead us through the next decade.

REFERENCES

1. Sande M, Ronald A. The academic alliance for AIDS care and prevention in Africa. Acad Med 2008;83(2):180–94.
2. Serwadda D, Magerwa RD, Sewankambo NK, et al. Slim disease: a new disease in Uganda and its association with HTLV-III infection. Lancet 1985;2(8460): 849–52.
3. Green EC, Halperin DT, Nantulya V, et al. Uganda's HIV prevention success: the role of sexual behavior change and the national response. AIDS Behav 2006; 10(4):335–46.
4. Slutkin G, Okware S, Naamara W, et al. How Uganda reversed its HIV epidemic. AIDS Behav 2006;10(4):351–60.
5. Parkhurst JO. Evidence, politics and Uganda's HIV success: moving forward with ABC and HIV prevention. J Int Dev February 22, 2010 [online].
6. Quinn T. The academic alliance for AIDS care and prevention in Africa. Hopkins HIV Rep 2001;13:1–3.
7. Scheld WM. One multidisciplinary approach to AIDS in Africa: the academic alliance for AIDS care and prevention in Africa in emerging infections. In: Scheld WM, Murray BE, Hughes JM, editors. Emerging Infections 4. Washington, DC: American Society of Microbiology; 2004. p. 83–99.
8. Ronald A, Sande M. HIV/AIDS care in Africa today. Clin Infect Dis 2005;40: 1045–8.
9. Wanyenze RK, Hahn JA, Liechty CA, et al. Linkage to HIV care and survival following inpatient HIV counseling and testing. AIDS Behav 2010 [online].
10. Petti CA, Polage CR, Quinn TC, et al. Laboratory medicine in Africa: a barrier to effective healthcare. Clin Infect Dis 2006;41:377–82.
11. Ronald A. Infectious diseases: a global human resource challenge. Curr Infect Dis Rep 2008;10(6):441–3.
12. Weaver MR, Nakitto C, Schneider G, et al. Measuring the outcomes of a comprehensive HIV care course: pilot test at the Infectious Diseases Institute, Kampala, Uganda. J Acquir Immune Defic Syndr 2006;43(3):293–303.

13. Wong M, Nakasujja N, Robertson K, et al. Prevalence of HIV dementia in an HIV clinic in sub-Saharan Africa. Neurology 2007;68:350–3.
14. Otiti-Sengeri J, Colebunders R, Kempen JH, et al. The prevalence and causes of visual loss among HIV-infected individuals. J Acquir Immune Defic Syndr 2010; 53:95–101.
15. Katwere M, Kambugu A, Piloya T, et al. Clinical presentation and aetiologies of acute or complicated headache among HIV-seropositive patients in a Ugandan clinic. J Int AIDS Soc 2009;12(1):21.
16. Ocama P, Katwere M, Piloya T, et al. The spectrum of liver diseases in HIV-infected individuals at an HIV treatment clinic in Kampala, Uganda. Afr Health Sci 2008;8(1):8–12.
17. Spacek LA, Shihab HM, Kamya MR, et al. Response to antiretroviral therapy in HIV-infected patients attending a public, urban clinic in Kampala, Uganda. Clin Infect Dis 2006;42:252–9.
18. Kambugu A, Meya DB, Rhein J, et al. Outcomes of cryptococcal meningitis in Uganda before and after the availability of highly active antiretroviral therapy. Clin Infect Dis 2008;46(11):1694–701.
19. Spacek LA, Shihab HM, Lutwama E, et al. Evaluation of a low-cost method, the Guana Easy CD4 assay, to enumerate CD4-positive lymphocyte counts in HIV-infected patients in the United States and Uganda. J Acquir Immune Defic Syndr 2006;41(5):607–10.
20. Lutwama F, Serwadda R, Mayanja-Kizza H, et al. Evaluation of Dynabeads and Cytospheres compared with flow cytometry to enumerate CD4+ T-cells in HIV-Infected Ugandans on antiretroviral therapy. J Acquir Immune Defic Syndr 2008;48(3):297–303.
21. DART Trial Team, Mugyenyi P, Walker AS, et al. Routine versus clinically driven laboratory monitoring of HIV antiretroviral therapy in Africa (DART): a randomized non-inferiority trial. Lancet 2010;375(9709):123–31.
22. Kamya MR, Mayanja-Kizza H, Kambugu A, et al. Predictors of long-term viral failure among Ugandan children and adults treated with antiretroviral therapy. J Acquir Immune Defic Syndr 2007;46(2):187–93.
23. Meya D, Spacek LA, Tibenderana H, et al. Development and evaluation of a clinical algorithm to monitor patients on antiretrovirals in resource-limited settings using adherence, clinical and CD4 cell count criteria. J Int AIDS Soc 2009; 12(1):3.
24. Castelnuovo B, Byakwaga H, Menten J, et al. Can response of a pruritic papular eruption to antiretroviral therapy be used as a clinical parameter to monitor virological outcomes? AIDS 2008;22(2):269–73.
25. Meya DB, Manabe YV, Castelnuovo B, et al. Cost-effectiveness of serum cryptococcal antigen screening to prevent deaths among HIV-infected persons with a CD4+ cell count ≤100 cells/microL who start HIV therapy in resource-limited settings. Clin Infect Dis 2010;51(4):448–55.
26. Lingappa JR, Baerten JM, Wald A, et al. Daily acyclovir for HIV-1 disease progression in people dually infected with HIV-1 and herpes simplex virus type 2: a randomized placebo-controlled trial. Lancet 2010;374(9717):824–33.
27. Celum C, Wald A, Lingappa JR, et al. Acyclovir and transmission of HIV-1 from persons infected with HIV-1 and HSV-2. N Engl J Med 2010;362(5):427–39.
28. Lamorde M, Byakikia-Kibwika P, Okaba-Kayom V, et al. Nevirapine pharmacokinetics when initiated at 200 mg or 400 mg daily in HIV-1 and tuberculosis co-infected Ugandan adults on rifampicin. J Antimicrob Chemother 2011;66(1):180–3.

29. Jacob ST, Moore CC, Banura P, et al. Severe sepsis in two Ugandan hospitals: a prospective observational study of management and outcomes in a predominantly HIV-1 infected population. PLoS One 2009;4(11):e7782.
30. Johnston C, Orem J, Okuku F, et al. Impact of HIV infection and Kaposi sarcoma on human herpes virus-8 mucosal replication and dissemination in Uganda. PLoS One 2009;4(1):e4222.
31. Sacktor N, Nakasuijja N, Skolasky RL, et al. HIV subtype D is associated with dementia compared with subtype A in immunosuppressed individuals at risk of cognitive impairment in Kampala, Uganda. Clin Infect Dis 2009;49(5):780–6.
32. Kalibala S, Kaleeba N. AIDS and community-based care in Uganda: the AIDS support organization, TASO. AIDS Care 1989;1(2):173–5.
33. Manabe YV, Jacob ST, Thomas D, et al. Resurrecting the triple threat: social responsibility in the context of global health research. Clin Infect Dis 2009; 48(10):1420–2.

Building a Global Health Education Network for Clinical Care and Research. The Benefits and Challenges of Distance Learning Tools. Lessons Learned from the Hopkins Center for Clinical Global Health Education

Robert C. Bollinger, MD, MPH*, Jane McKenzie-White, MAS, Amita Gupta, MD, MHS

KEYWORDS

• Distance learning • mHealth • Research • Clinical • Education • Global health

Tell me and I forget. Show me and I remember. Involve me and I understand.
Chinese Proverb

Expanding the capacity for clinical care and health research is a global priority and a global challenge. In disenfranchised communities facing the largest burden of disease, whether they are in rural Africa or urban United States, there is a great need for more well-trained, competent, and dedicated health care providers. In addition, globalization has necessitated that an understanding of global health issues is a requirement for all health care providers, whether they be community health workers in rural Uganda, private practitioners in Mumbai or Los Angeles, or faculty at Johns

Disclosure: See last page of article.

Center for Clinical Global Health Education, Johns Hopkins School of Medicine, Johns Hopkins University, Phipps 540, 600 North Wolfe Street, Baltimore, MD 21287, USA
* Corresponding author.
E-mail address: rcb@jhmi.edu

Infect Dis Clin N Am 25 (2011) 385–398
doi:10.1016/j.idc.2011.02.006
id.theclinics.com
0891-5520/11/$ – see front matter

Hopkins Medical School. Resource-limited communities also require a greater capacity for and ownership of their own health research priorities and programs. Meeting these pressing needs for human capacity building in health care and research requires additional resources and innovation. Traditional approaches to clinical and research education are important and necessary but not sufficient to achieve the scale and pace of human capacity building required. Distance learning programs, that include mHealth as well as other information technology (IT) platforms and tools, can provide unique, timely, cost-effective, and valuable opportunities to expand access to training, clinical care support and strategic information for clinicians and researchers, throughout the world.

Advances and investments in IT are providing many new tools for delivering and accessing information, as well as for learning. These tools and new IT infrastructure are rapidly becoming available in developing countries and resource-limited communities around the world, providing new opportunities for clinical and research capacity building initiatives. Effective distance learning programs have been developed, and they use multiple tools in the IT toolbox to optimize their capacity building and teaching. In addition to providing optimal content to address the learning objectives of specific training programs, it is also important to strategically choose the optimal tools to deliver and access this content, as well as to recognize the limitations of distance learning and to rigorously evaluate the impact of any training program. These steps are essential before major investment of resources and time that are required for the scale-up and large-scale implementation of distance education programs to expand global health man power and capacity.

The Johns Hopkins Center for Clinical Global Health Education (CCGHE) was established in 2005 to provide access to high-quality training to health care providers in resource-limited settings. The CCGHE made a strategic decision to develop, use, and evaluate distance learning platforms to achieve its mission. In the initial years of this new program, several lessons have been learned that may be helpful to other programs considering the use of distance learning programs to expand global health clinical and research capacity.

WHAT IS DISTANCE LEARNING?

Distance learning involves the strategic use of multiple IT tools to teach and learn. Distance learning programs also typically use IT tools to evaluate the impact of the programs. The distance learning toolbox includes multiple platforms to interact with and to access and deploy information that may be important for clinicians and researchers. In some cases, the most effective training content can be text based or image based. Audio, video, and interactive formats, including simulation platforms, can also be used. Multimedia content and large amounts of data can be shared in very portable formats, including digital videodiscs, CD-ROMs, CDs, thumb drives. Web sites, portals, and local area networks can also store and deploy multimedia content. Availability of reliable fiber or wireless networks can support use of e-mail, web streaming, videoconferencing, chat rooms, social networks, cell phones, smart devices, and other interactive platforms to facilitate training. These formats can be used for live group-learning experiences, often referred to as synchronous learning formats. In many cases, asynchronous platforms, including e-mail, online forums, and social networking sites, can be very efficient and effective methods to facilitate faculty-student interactions and group learning. Many of these tools are well known and used in developed countries, where distance learning is more widely established. The CCGHE has used multiple tools in this toolbox, as well as developed new tools and approaches to optimize our mission to support health care providers in very remote communities.

PROVIDERS IN RESOURCE-LIMITED SETTINGS USE THE WEB TO LEARN

When the CCGHE was launched, a simple Web site was one of the first distance learning tools developed and used, in which content specifically relevant to providers in resource-limited settings was made available.[1] Initially, these tools were simply text, PDF files, or Web links of key best practices and guidelines from governments and organizations such as the Centers for Disease Control and Prevention, World Health Organization, United Nations AIDS, International AIDS Society. In addition, links to live and recorded Web casts of weekly Infectious Diseases Grand Rounds from Johns Hopkins were made available. Within a matter of months, the number of visits to this Web site quickly increased to more than 500,000 hits per month from more than 100 different countries, including many countries in Africa, Asia, and Latin America (**Fig. 1**). This rapid demonstration of interest and demand for clinical training content were surprising, given that this demand was generated without any significant public advertisement or effort by the CCGHE to announce the launch of its Web site or program. In addition to the demonstration that providers from resource-limited communities in Africa, Asia, and Latin America use the Web to learn, the authors' early experience with the CCGHE Web site demonstrated the power of the Web to rapidly share information around the world.

DISTANCE LEARNING IS FEASIBLE AND COST-EFFECTIVE FOR RESOURCE-LIMITED SETTINGS

One of the first CCGHE initiatives to develop a full distance learning course was for human immunodeficiency virus (HIV) health care providers in Zambia. There are several learning management systems (LMSs) available to develop and deploy distance learning courses. From its inception, the CCGHE has made a strategic decision to use less-expensive open-source tools for the training programs, whenever possible. Therefore, the first distance learning course used the open-source LMS

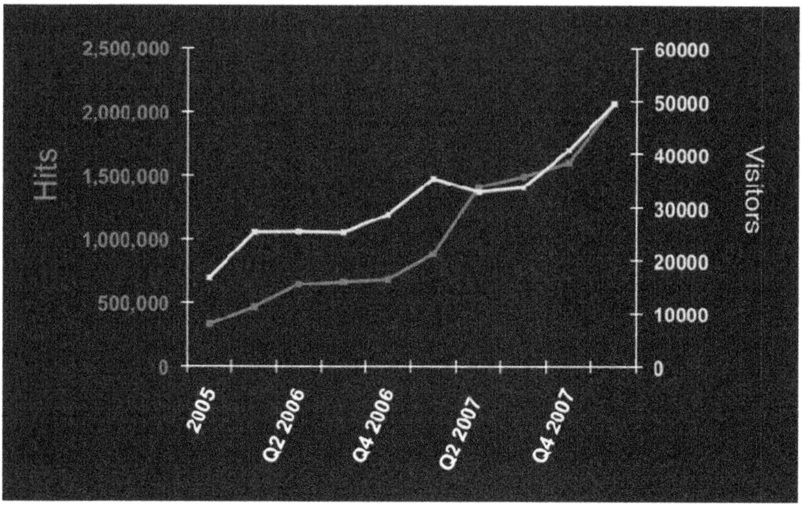

Fig. 1. Initial CCGHE Web site activity.

program called Moodle.[2] The HIV clinical care course for Zambia consisted of 21 recorded lectures by Hopkins and Zambian experts, which were formatted into 5 modules and made available on the Web and CD-ROM, for participants without reliable Web access. The course was delivered over a 6-week period and included a weekly live faculty Web chat and online discussion forum. Course learning objectives were reenforced through case discussions, as well as questions/answer (Q&A) sessions with the faculty. To the authors' knowledge, this was the first distance learning course ever offered in Zambia. Despite great efforts by collaborating organizations in Zambia, it was initially very difficult to convince students to participate in this first course. Reasons for this reluctance to participate in a distance learning course included a healthy skepticism about the reliability of Internet access in Zambia that is required for the low-bandwidth live faculty chats, course registration, and knowledge testing. In addition, there was uncertainty about the benefit of participating in a distance learning course related to HIV clinical care, and there was also a concern that providers in Zambia would not participate in a free training course that does not incentivize them with payment for their participation.

Despite a challenging initial launch, the course was successfully deployed and included the live synchronized chats. The value and feasibility of a distance learning course format, even in a setting such as Zambia with very limited Internet connectivity, were evidenced by the great demand for this course and by the successful online participation of Zambian clinicians. A particularly notable demonstration of feasibility was the success of one live online session led by a Hopkins faculty member from Dhaka, Bangladesh, linked to the course participants in Zambia. Within 1 month of completion of the first HIV clinical care course with 83 registered participants, Zambian colleagues requested that the course be redeployed, and more than 281 students registered for the second session of this course. An additional 499 students registered for the third session of this course. In addition to demonstrating to the CCGHE and its partners in Zambia that distance learning is a feasible and valued training format for clinicians in resource-limited settings, this Zambian course demonstrated the cost-effectiveness of a distance learning format.

As shown in **Fig. 2**, the initial cost of recording and developing this course for the first 83 registered students was $1204 per student. Because recurring costs for the second and third sessions of this course were much less, the cost per student was ultimately reduced to $171. Therefore, the per-student cost of conducting a 6-week 21-lecture distance learning course, delivered to approximately 900 Zambian clinicians, by Zambian and US faculty experts was significantly less than that of HIV training courses offered in Zambia.[3] In addition, the distance learning format permitted a more flexible schedule for students who were able to participate in this course without interrupting their normal work schedule. Although the feedback from the course evaluation completed by Zambian participants was extremely positive and significant knowledge gains were demonstrated through knowledge test scores, there was no opportunity to compare the impact of this online course with that of other more-standard training formats. This early experience highlighted the need for resources and opportunity to properly evaluate any training program, particularly those using new distance-education technology.

DISTANCE LEARNING IS EMPOWERING AND FACILITATES SOUTH-SOUTH CAPACITY BUILDING

One of the most successful and most sustainable CCGHE programs was initiated in 2006 in collaboration with colleagues at the Addis Ababa University (AAU) in Ethiopia.

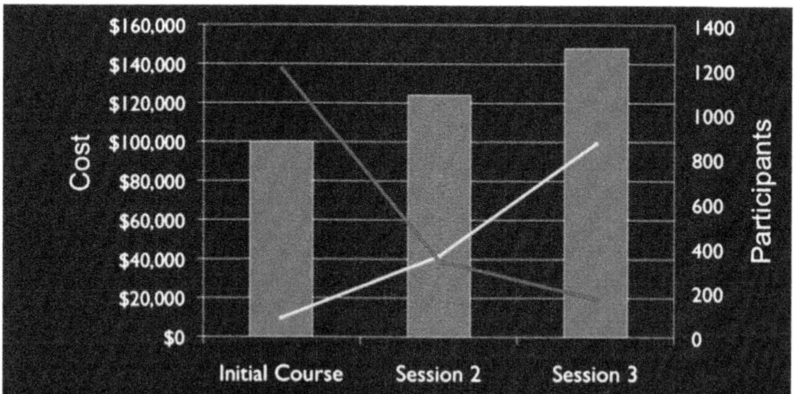

	Jan-Feb 2008	Sept-Oct 08	Feb-March 09
Session Cost	$100,000	$24,000	$24,000
Total Cost	$100,000	$124,000	$148,000
Session Trainees	83	281	499
Total Trainees	83	364	863
Cost per Trainee	$1204	$341	$171

Fig. 2. Cost and scale of online HIV clinical care course in Zambia.

The format for this program began as live videoconference-supported presentations and discussions of clinical cases of patients with HIV infection by faculty and students from the AAU, Hopkins, Mayo Clinic, and University of South Carolina. The initiation of this program was also made possible through the support of several other sponsors and stakeholders, including the US President's Emergency Plan for AIDS Relief and the World Bank Global Development Learning Network (GDLN), who provided access to their videoconferencing facility in Addis Ababa to launch this program. Again, this was the first time that this type of distance learning format had been undertaken in Ethiopia, and, not surprisingly, there was considerable early skepticism about its feasibility, value, and sustainability. In the early phase of this program, 20 to 30 busy faculty were expected to drive a long distance every other Friday afternoon, from AAU to the Civil Service College in Addis Ababa, the location of the GDLN facility, to participate in this program. At each session, 2 to 3 clinical cases are presented and discussed by the participating faculty. These case discussions were recorded and made available through live and archived Web casts, as well as burned on CD-ROMs and shipped to Ethiopia for distribution around the country to providers without reliable Internet or access to the videoconferencing facility.

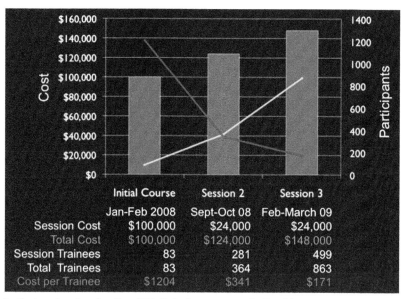

The early case discussions were notable for the US faculty providing much of the discussion and input. However, within a very short period, the faculty in Ethiopia took ownership and leadership of this program. Now, 4 years after a skeptical and difficult start to the program, more than 200 case discussions have been recorded and distributed throughout Ethiopia, and clinicians throughout the world have benefited by viewing these excellent discussions online. The program was such a success that the AAU has now built its own state-of-the-art videoconferencing facility in their medical school auditorium, expanding participation to many more faculty and students. In addition, 2 more Ethiopian medical schools have built similar facilities and are now actively participating in these case conferences, which continue to be broadcasted throughout the world. The recent global availability of the infrastructure for videoconferencing is a tremendous opportunity to initiate similar programs and is a particularly valuable platform for learning in the context of clinical case discussions, clinical consultations, and group learning.[4] The success of the CCGHE program in Ethiopia has led directly to the recent initiation of similar videoconference clinical education programs in other countries, including India and Palestine.[5–7]

Another demonstration of the value of distance learning to support south-south collaboration is a recent CCGHE course focused on diagnosis, treatment, and prevention of tuberculosis. This was an in-depth, comprehensive, 6-week, modular course, with 25 prerecorded lectures and live videoconference-supported activities that engaged faculty from the United States and South Africa as well as faculty and 235 students from India and Pakistan in a vibrant and interactive learning experience that resulted in well-documented improvements in knowledge for the students. This course, supported by the Fogarty International Training Program, deployed the 25 lectures and other course materials on CD-ROMs. Students completed online precourse and postcourse knowledge assessments, as well as course evaluations. In addition, 11 live videoconference discussion sessions were scheduled, linking faculty and students at BJ Medical College and National AIDS Research Institute in India, Indus Hospital in Pakistan, and Johns Hopkins in Baltimore, Maryland. To accommodate participants unable to participate in the videoconferences, an Internet link was established to view the live Web cast, with the ability to ask questions. In addition, an asynchronous Q&A discussion forum was available on the course Web site, in which participants post questions at any time for the faculty and fellow participants. Faculty monitored the forum and responded to questions posted within 36 to 72 hours. In addition, links to the recorded videoconference sessions were posted in both low- and high-bandwidth formats and accessible to participants through the Web site. The median correct score for the pretests was 66% compared with 86% for the posttest, and 95% of students completing the posttest received a score of more than 70%, which was the cutoff for the certification of competence with the material. More than 90% of the respondents to the course evaluation "agreed" or "strongly agreed" that the course objectives and expectations were clearly defined, the course was organized in a way that facilitated learning, the lectures were of high quality and of an appropriate length, the content was applicable to their practice setting, and they would recommend the course to a colleague and would take a similar course again.

DISTANCE LEARNING AND mHEALTH TOOLS CAN SUPPORT TASK SHIFTING

A critical challenge to improvements in global health is the limited number of trained physicians, nurses, and other health professionals. This health man power gap is a well-recognized challenge, and several public and private stakeholders have begun to address this need.[8] As illustrated earlier, strategic use of distance learning tools can support these efforts to train high-level providers and to expand the capacity of health institutions. However, in most resource-limited settings, low-level health care providers with limited access to professional training provide much of the health care in the communities. Providing access to training and clinical care support to these community health workers is also often challenged by rural and remote practice settings as well as by the financial and opportunity costs of traditional training programs that typically require providers to leave their practices and communities to receive training. Novel use of distance learning tools, particularly wireless mHealth platforms, provides opportunities to scale-up health care capacity building initiatives and to address the training needs of community health workers and other providers in remote communities.

The development of a recent distance learning adult male circumcision course in Uganda illustrates how distance learning can support scale-up of high-priority specialized training. The Rakai Health Sciences Program (RHSP) is internationally known for its research demonstrating that adult male circumcision can reduce the risk of HIV acquisition.[9] This demonstration has led to large-scale programs to expand the training of medical personnel in this procedure.[10] The RHSP conducts an excellent circumcision training program for providers from around Africa. However, the impact of this program and other similar programs is limited by the time and expense required. To be certified in the RHSP course, a trainee typically travels to Rakai for 2 weeks to participate in lectures and demonstrations and to perform an average of 20 supervised circumcisions.[11] To increase the efficiency, reduce the cost, and increase the scale of the RHSP circumcision training program, the CCGHE created the Adult Male Circumcision Training eLearning Program, which was developed by the experts involved in the RHSP. This course provides instruction on the required steps to perform the dorsal slit surgery and all the necessary preoperative and postoperative screening and care. Packaged for CD-ROM use, this e-Learning program and its knowledge assessment test can be used as pretraining material and/or as a refresher and reference after hands-on training. The program is organized into 5 sections: (1) preoperative considerations, (2) surgical preparations, (3) the dorsal slit surgical procedure, (4) postoperative care, and (5) management of complications. The program also includes 2 hours of lectures, high-definition video demonstrations, and interactive exercises. The purpose of this e-Learning course is to allow trainees to successfully complete the course before coming to Rakai, where the expectation is that trainees will be better prepared for hands-on training, and the time required to achieve certification could then be significantly less than the current 2 weeks. This upgrade would lead to improved efficiency, increased scale, and reduced cost of the current RHSP circumcision training program. This example illustrates that distance learning tools are not a replacement for hands-on, bedside, or face-to-face training; rather, these tools can be coordinated with more-standard training platforms to increase the overall capacity of the existing training programs.

mHealth programs, taking advantage of the expanding wireless infrastructure, are an increasingly important component of distance learning initiatives. mHealth interventions are particularly valuable for providing training and clinical care support to patients, low-level health workers, and other providers, using and delivering community-based and home care health services. To expand access to training to providers in rural African community settings, the CCGHE developed a secure, highly flexible and adaptable, open-source mHealth application called the electronic Mobile Open-Source Comprehensive Health Application (eMOCHA). This application, which was selected as a finalist for the 2010 Vodafone Wireless Innovation Award program, is designed to leverage mobile phones to assist health programs, researchers, providers, and patients to improve communication, education, patient care, and data collection.

eMOCHA synergizes the power of (1) mobile technology, (2) Android-supported devices, (3) video and audio files, and (4) a server-based application to analyze and GPS (global positioning system) map large amounts of data, implement interactive multimedia training, and streamline data collection and analyses. eMOCHA runs not only on all Android devices, smart phones, and tablets but also on regular cell phones, with the capacity to send and receive data through a Web-based interface, using toll-free SMS (short messaging service) (**Fig. 3**). eMOCHA projects are currently being deployed and evaluated in a wide range of health care, public health, and research programs in Uganda, Afghanistan, and the United States, with additional projects

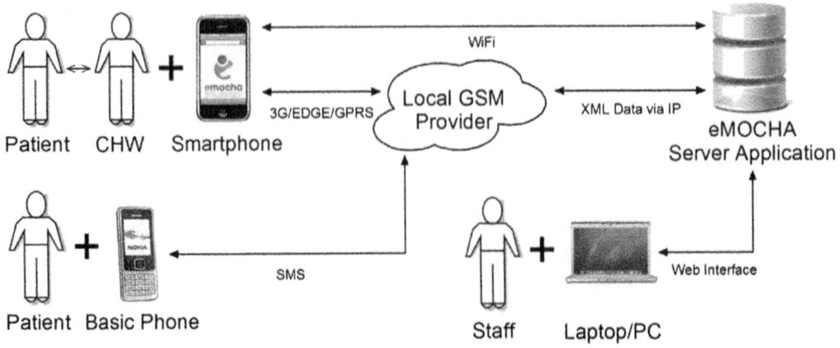

Fig. 3. eMOCHA mHealth application for clinical training and care support. 3G, third generation; EDGE, enhanced data rates for GSM evolution; GPRS, general packet radio service; GSM, global system for mobile communications; IP, internet protocol; PC, personal computer.

under development in Central America, India, Bangladesh, and Ethiopia. These diverse projects include community and home-based strategies to optimize HIV counseling and testing, HIV treatment adherence, tuberculosis diagnosis and treatment, malaria prevention and treatment, maternal and child health, reduction of intravenous drug use, management of chronic diseases, and prevention of domestic violence. mHealth platforms, such as eMOCHA, can provide unique opportunities to empower health care providers, even in the most remote locations, with point-of-care strategic training and clinical care support. The rapid growth and potential of mHealth programs to address global health priorities has led recently to new initiatives to support the development and evaluation of these innovative tools, including programs supported by the Gates Foundation Grand Challenges,[12] The Rockefeller Foundation,[13] the mHealth Alliance.[14] However, as with most other uses of technology to improve health, there are limited data demonstrating that mHealth interventions improve health outcomes or clinical practice, particularly in resource-limited settings. The deployment of wireless devices and applications by health programs is rapidly expanding, despite the lack of good public health impact data to support their widespread deployment. The mHealth field seems to be following the "ready, fire, aim" strategy, highlighting the urgent need for rigorous and well-designed evaluations of these initiatives.

DISTANCE LEARNING EMPOWERS AND FACILITATES SOUTH-NORTH GLOBAL HEALTH CAPACITY BUILDING

In February 2010, a new global health course was offered for all first year Johns Hopkins medical students, which took advantage of the new distance learning capacity to connect medical students in Baltimore with students and faculty in Uganda, Ethiopia, Pakistan, and India. The purpose of this course was to introduce basic global health concepts to first year medical students. This course shows not only that distance learning can support unique educational experiences that leverage technology and global connectivity but also the power of group learning and "South-North" capacity building. The course was organized into 4 themes, with each day beginning with the presentation, discussion, and comparison of 2 representative clinical cases of the same health problem from 2 very different settings (**Table 1**). The course was very successful and received strong favorable feedback from students at Hopkins and from the other 4 partner institutions. The ability to interact with each other through

Table 1
Hopkins medical students global health course live videoconference case discussions

Day	Theme	Clinical Cases	Partner Institutes
1	Maternal health	High-risk pregnancy in Baltimore and Addis Ababa	AAU, Black Lion Hospital
2	Child health	Pediatric pneumonia in Baltimore and Kampala	Makerere University, Mulago Hospital
3	Emerging diseases	MDR-TB in Baltimore and Karachi	Indus Hospital
4	Chronic diseases	Coronary artery disease in Baltimore and Pune	BJ Medical College, Sassoon Hospital

Abbreviation: MDR-TB, multidrug-resistant tuberculosis.

live videoconferencing enriched the global health learning experience.[15] However, the use of this high-tech distance learning platform also provided many wonderful opportunities to discuss the limitations of technology. The Hopkins students, who were attentively engaged by their open laptops during the class, were challenged with questions about why they needed to use their cell phones and laptops during the class from the Ethiopian students, who were focused and engaged in the discussion without the help of these devices (**Fig. 4**). During the discussion of 2 pediatric pneumococcal pneumonia cases, the Ugandan medical students asked the Hopkins students whether they were taught to use stethoscopes; the diagnostic workup of the child in Baltimore was described and included a computed tomographic scan of the chest, as well as multiple subspecialty consultations and a 14-day hospital course, whereas the child from Uganda, with the same diagnosis, the same antibiotic treatment, and the same successful clinical outcome was diagnosed with an excellent physical examination and a chest radiograph. In the latter case, the child was also discharged home from the hospital after 2 inpatient days with a prescription of oral antibiotics. The use of distance learning technology to facilitate these discussions of global health issues ironically provided a tremendously valuable opportunity for the Hopkins students to learn from their colleagues in Ethiopia, Uganda, Pakistan, and India about the limits of technology as well as the importance of professionalism and a good physical examination.

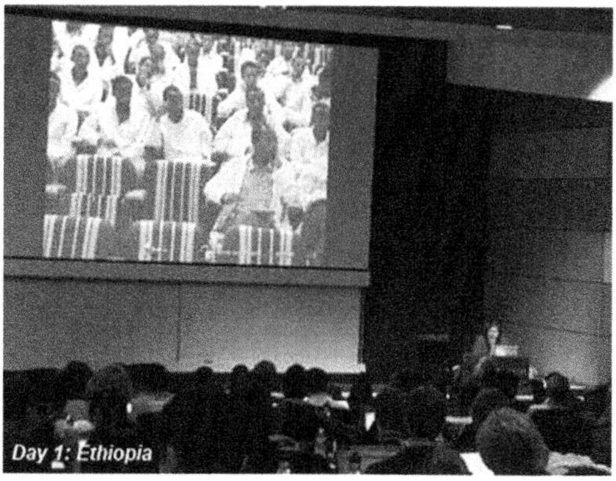

Fig. 4. Hopkins first year medical students global health case discussion with AAU and Black Lion Hospital in Ethiopia.

DISTANCE LEARNING CAN AND MUST BE EVALUATED

Online learning has been widely used for education in the United States and other developed country settings, where its effectiveness has been demonstrated.[16] Although distance education is also increasingly supporting the training of students in resource-limited settings, evaluations of the impact and acceptance of distance learning platforms in such settings are limited. To better understand the potential value of distance education to expand health research capacity, the CCGHE undertook a randomized study comparing online with on-site (ie, face to face) delivery of courses in 2 distinct domains relevant for international health research: Biostatistics and Research Ethics (Aggarwal R, Gupte N, Kass N, et al. Distance learning to build international health research capacity: a randomized study of online vs on-site training. Submitted for publication). The authors' hypothesis was that both on-site and online course formats would lead to similar gains in knowledge for students, for both content domains.

A total of 58 Indian scientist volunteers were randomly assigned to 1 of 2 arms. Volunteers in arm 1 attended a 3.5-day on-site course in Biostatistics and completed a 3.5-week online course in Research Ethics. Volunteers in arm 2 attended a 3.5-week online course in Biostatistics and 3.5-day on-site course in Research Ethics. For the 2 course formats, learning objectives and knowledge tests were identical and course contents were similar. The improvement in knowledge was assessed immediately and 3 months after course completion and compared with baseline. Baseline characteristics were similar in both arms. As shown in **Fig. 5**, immediate median gains in knowledge scores were similar between the on-site and online platforms for both Biostatistics and Research Ethics. The increase in knowledge gain was sustained 3 months after completion of the courses and remained similar for the on-site and online formats.

In summary, evaluation of this distance education program in India demonstrated that online and on-site training formats led to marked and similar improvements of knowledge in Biostatistics and Research Ethics. This program, combined with logistic and cost advantages of online training, may make online courses particularly useful for expanding health research capacity in resource-limited settings. The authors' experience also demonstrates that precourse and postcourse knowledge assessments, as well as student course evaluations can be easily deployed and monitored, even for learners in remote areas. In addition to interactive learning tools deployed online, wireless devices can also be used to both deliver and evaluate training programs. Although randomized study designs are not always feasible or necessary for evaluation of distance education programs, rigorous evaluations should be a responsibility and priority for health programs that use them.

DISTANCE LEARNING LIMITATIONS AND BENEFITS

Distance learning tools are designed to supplement and support capacity building programs and not to replace other more-traditional training platforms. As with any education strategy, distance learning tools have limitations. The optimal use of these tools requires an understanding of the required infrastructure and technological support. Structural barriers such as limited fiber networks, bandwidth, and wireless network architecture, as well as lack of access to computers can be important barriers to the effective use of distance learning technology. In some cases, students lack the experience and training required to use the technologies. Whereas cell phones are ubiquitous and may be optimal tools for many settings, many individuals may be unfamiliar with computers. These challenges require any capacity building program using

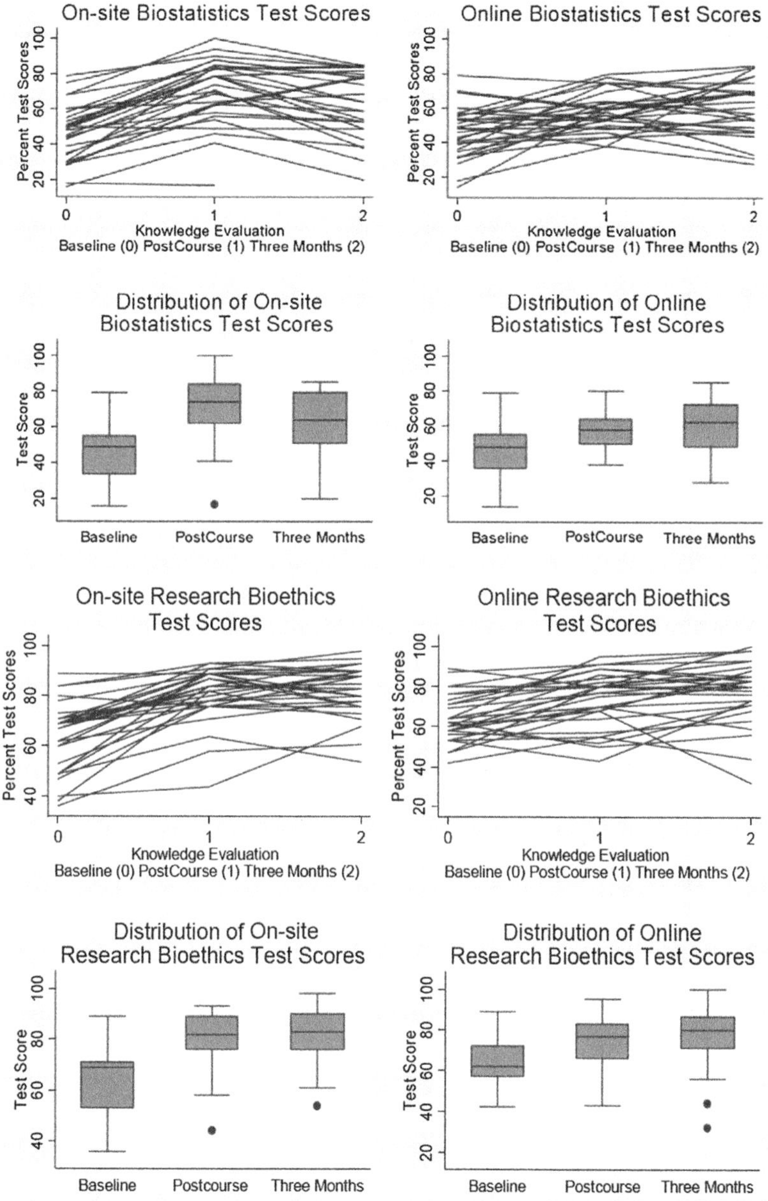

Fig. 5. Comparison of knowledge gain between online and on-site courses in Biostatistics and Research Ethics.

distance learning platforms to have a clear understanding of which tools work optimally in their own settings. In many settings, distance learning may provide access to basic information, but high-level training, particularly clinical or laboratory skills, still requires hands-on training, and face-to-face mentorship or group interactions. In addition, effective health care delivery requires that providers and patients develop trust and familiarity with each other. It would be a mistake for technology to replace or interfere with the human-to-human interactions that are so important for students to experience and learn.

Despite these important limitations, when carefully designed and implemented, distance learning tools provide a unique opportunity to expand access to training and clinical care support for resource-limited providers and communities (**Box 1**). The flexibility of these tools can prioritize important local competencies and training gaps. The CCGHE experience suggests that distance learning tools can rapidly deliver new information and adapt to changing local needs. They are feasible to implement, even in very remote communities in Asia, Africa, and Latin America. In general, the lower cost of deployment increases the accessibility and scalability of training programs, making distance learning more cost-effective and sustainable for resource-constrained communities. Distance learning is also a "green" technology that limits the need for travel for both learners and trainers. In contrast to live workshops or face-to-face lectures, distance learning also allows capturing the very best available training, as well as for more consistent delivery of the highest-quality training content to many different settings. Interactive distance learning platforms also allow for content delivery to adapt to the understanding and experience of learners, leading to broad utility for students with diverse literacy, experience, and prior education. In addition, as opposed to more traditional education strategies that "push" the content to learners, distance education is a "pull" platform that requires learners to access and use the content. Therefore, distance learners are active learners and only use and demand content that is valuable to them. This provides additional incentive to education programs that use distance learning technology to optimize their content.

Distance learning can, therefore, empower local providers and, perhaps, limit "brain drain." The flexibility and convenience of distance learning tools allow providers to access training and clinical care support at their point of care, own homes, or local communities. Typically, they can also more easily control the timing of their training. In summary, distance learning programs empower the learner and limit the need for providers to leave their communities to access high-quality training.

The future scale and acceptability of distance learning tools to support global health education will ultimately depend on the clear demonstration of impact and value. There is a great need for rigorous evaluation and monitoring of distance learning programs. As with any training program, distance education programs must lead to improved clinical practice and improved health for the communities and patients. Although technology and innovation lead to greater opportunities for distance

Box 1
Benefits of distance learning programs

- Flexible and feasible for most resource-limited settings
- Can prioritize local needs
- Lower cost for deployment, scalability, and sustainability
- Lower opportunity costs for learners
- "Green" technology
- Active empowered learners
- Consistent delivery of highest-quality content
- Adaptable to diverse learner experience, education, and literacy

learning, in communities around the world, there is also an opportunity and responsibility to properly evaluate and monitor these programs.

DISCLOSURES

Dr Bollinger's research and education programs have been supported by grants from the National Institutes of Health, the US Centers for Disease Control, the Bill and Melinda Gates Foundation, the President's Emergency Plan for AIDS Relief (PEPFAR). Ms McKenzie-White's education programs are supported by grants from the National Institutes of Health. Dr Gupta's research and education programs are supported by grants from the National Institutes of Health and the Gilead Foundation. The education programs of the Johns Hopkins Center for Clinical Global Health Education have been supported by BASF; Brayton Wilbur Foundation; The Indira Foundation; John and Amy Weinberg Foundation; Lazard Freres & Co LLC; Otto Haas Charitable Trust; Schering-Plough; Wilbur-Ellis Company Foundation; Northwater Foundation; HB Fuller Company Foundation; Nova Chemicals; Auxillium Pharmaceuticals Inc; Black Enterprise Magazine; Dow Chemical Company Foundation; GlaxoSmithKline; Nalco Foundation; The VF Foundation; the William Penn Foundation; Astellas Pharma; Boehringer Ingelheim Pharmaceuticals, Inc; Pfizer, Inc; Gilead Sciences, Inc; and Tibotec Therapeutics.

REFERENCES

1. Johns Hopkins Center for Clinical Global Health Education. 2010. Available at: http://www.ccghe.jhmi.edu/ccg/index.asp. Accessed November 19, 2010.
2. Moodle Course Management System. 2010. Available at: http://moodle.org/. Accessed November 19, 2010.
3. Huddart J, Furth R, Lyons J. The Zambia HIV/AIDS Workforce Study: preparing for scale-up. April 2004 Report of the Quality Assurance Project (QAP). U.S. Agency for International Development (USAID). Contract Number GPH-C-00-02-00004-00.
4. Johns Hopkins Center for Clinical Global Health Education. Global vision-delivering web-based education around the world. 2010. Available at: http://www.ccghe.net/video/1GlobalVision.html. Accessed November 19, 2010.
5. Johns Hopkins Center for Clinical Global Health Education. HIV clinical care discussions in Ethiopia. 2010. Available at: http://www.ccghe.jhmi.edu/CCG/distance/HIV_Courses/Ethiopiaart.asp. Accessed November 19, 2010.
6. Johns Hopkins Center for Clinical Global Health Education. HIV clinical care discussions in India. 2010. Available at: http://www.ccghe.jhmi.edu/CCG/distance/HIV_Discussions_India/. Accessed November 19, 2010.
7. Johns Hopkins Center for Clinical Global Health Education. Continuing Medical Education Course for family practitioners in Palestine. 2010. Available at: http://moodle.ccghe.net/course/view.php?id=48. Accessed November 19, 2010.
8. World Health Organization. Global recommendations and guidelines on task shifting. Geneva (Switzerland): World Health Organization; 2007.
9. Gray RH, Kigozi G, Serwadda D, et al. Male circumcision for HIV prevention in men in Rakai, Uganda: a randomised trial. Lancet 2007;369(9562):657–66.
10. World Health Organization and Joint United Nations Programme on HIV/AIDS. Operational guidance for scaling up male circumcision services for HIV prevention. 2008. Available at: http://www.malecircumcision.org/programs/documents/MC_OpGuideFINAL_web.pdf. Accessed November 19, 2010.

11. Kiggundu V, Watya S, Kigozi G, et al. The number of procedures required to achieve optimal competency with male circumcision: findings from a randomized trial in Rakai, Uganda. BJU Int 2009;104(4):529–32.
12. Bill and Melinda Gates Foundation. Grand Challenges in Global Health Round 5. Create low-cost cell phone-based applications for priority global health conditions. March 2010. Available at: http://www.grandchallenges.org/MeasureHealthStatus/Topics/CellPhoneApps/Pages/Round5.aspx. Accessed November 19, 2010.
13. The Rockefeller Foundation. From Silos to Systems: an overview of eHealth's Transformative Power. Rockefeller Foundation Report/Bellagio Center Conference Series January 13, 2010. Available at: http://www.rockefellerfoundation.org/news/publications/from-silos-systems-overview-ehealth. Accessed November 19, 2010.
14. mHealth Alliance. Available at: http://www.mhealthalliance.org/. Accessed November 19, 2010.
15. Johns Hopkins Center for Clinical Global Health Education. Global Health Course for Medical Students. Emerging infections case discussion: Indus Hospital in Karachi and Johns Hopkins in Baltimore. March 2010. Available at: http://moodle.ccghe.net/media/IndusHospital.mp4. Accessed November 19, 2010.
16. US Department of Education, Office of Planning, Evaluation and Policy Development. Evaluation of evidence-based practices in online learning: a meta-analysis and review of online learning studies. Washington, DC, 2009. Available at: http://www.ed.gov/about/offices/list/opepd/ppss/reports.html. Accessed November 19, 2010.

Printed and bound by CPI Group (UK) Ltd, Croydon, CR0 4YY

03/10/2024

01040458-0014

The Afya Bora Consortium: An Africa-US Partnership to Train Leaders in Global Health

Carey Farquhar, MD, MPH[a,*], Neal Nathanson, MD[b], Consortium Working Group[1]

KEYWORDS

• Global health • Africa • Education • Training • Research • HIV/AIDS • Leadership • Partnership

In the last 10 years, the sub-Saharan African AIDS epidemic has been a major stimulus for rapidly increasing investments in newly developed and existing health programs. These burgeoning programs have generated an increasing demand for African leaders in global health. The largest program is the President's Emergency Program for AIDS Relief (PEPFAR), launched in 2003. Many other health programs have recently been launched in Africa, supported by national and international agencies, such as the Global Fund, the Global Alliance for Vaccines and Immunization, United Nation (UN) AIDS, the World Health Organization (WHO), the World Bank, and others. In addition, there is a panoply of health programs supported by foundations, private philanthropy, and other nongovernment organizations (NGOs). It has been estimated that there are more than 1000 NGOs operating in Kenya alone.[1]

Rapid expansion of these programs has created a need for African medical, nursing, and public health professionals who can design, manage, and evaluate large health programs. Similar growth in the research arena has resulted in an increased demand for trained investigators to lead complex research programs. At present, too many programs depend on expatriates who have been recruited because of the shortage

This work was supported by a supplement to Grant No. D43TW000007-22S3 from the Fogarty International Center of the U.S. National Institutes of Health.

[a] Division of Allergy and Infectious Disease, Departments of Medicine and Epidemiology and Global Health, University of Washington, 325 Ninth Avenue, Box 359909, Seattle, WA 98104, USA
[b] Global Health Programs, School of Medicine, University of Pennsylvania, 1007 Blockley Hall, 423 Guardian Drive, Philadelphia, PA 19104-6021, USA
[1] See Acknowledgments for membership of the Working Group.
* Corresponding author.
E-mail address: cfarq@u.washington.edu

of local professionals with appropriate skills. Several independent groups have recognized the need for African leadership and have called for new training initiatives.[2–4] The Afya Bora Consortium is a response to this call to action. This consortium is founded on the premise that a consortium of African and international health institutions can pool resources to develop an innovative, robust, and sustainable program to train future leaders in global health. The authors present this interdisciplinary experiential approach to leadership training as a model that could be adapted to meet the needs of other regions and expanded to include additional institutional partnerships.

HISTORY OF THE AFYA BORA CONSORTIUM

The vision for a consortium of US and African institutions dedicated to building leadership capacity in global health was born in May 2008 when a group of US faculty members, who are leaders of global health programs at their 4 institutions, met in Washington, DC. Each university has an established "twinning" relationship with an African academic health center, and all 8 institutions have both schools of medicine and nursing and many have schools of public health (**Table 1**). As a next step, it was decided to convene a workshop for an exploration of needs and opportunities.[5–7]

In April 2009, representatives of the 8 institutions met at a 2-day workshop in Nairobi, Kenya. After much collegial discussion, the group decided to create a Consortium to develop a 2-year Fellowship. This Fellowship was designed for medical, nursing, and public health professionals who had recently completed their training and were judged to have leadership potential. A 1-year fellowship and individual short modules for in-service training were also included in response to requests for options that would meet a broader array of leadership training needs. The following month, the proposal was presented to potential sponsors at a meeting in Washington, DC. A 1-year planning grant was funded by the Fogarty International Center of the US National Institutes of Health, beginning in September 2009.

This Africa-US partnership has been named the Afya Bora (Swahili for "Better Health") Consortium. At a meeting in Nairobi, Kenya, in January 2010, it was decided that a 1-year Pilot program of the Fellowship should be conducted to test its components, evaluate outcomes, and prepare for a sustainable program. In July 2010, a grant proposal for a Pilot program of the Afya Bora Leadership Fellowship was presented, a summary of which is the subject of this article.

Table 1
The Afya Bora Consortium institutions and health sciences schools

Country	African-US Partner Institutions	Medical School	Nursing School	Public Health School
Uganda	Makerere University	Yes	Yes	Yes
United States	Johns Hopkins University	Yes	Yes	Yes
Tanzania	Muhimbili University of Health and Allied Sciences	Yes	Yes	Yes
United States	University of California San Francisco	Yes	Yes	Yes
Botswana	University of Botswana	Yes	Yes	No
United States	University of Pennsylvania	Yes	Yes	No
Kenya	University of Nairobi	Yes	Yes	Yes
United States	University of Washington	Yes	Yes	Yes

DESCRIPTION OF THE PILOT PROGRAM

The Pilot program is a scaled-down version of the full Afya Bora Fellowship, designed to "beta test" the key elements of the full fellowship within the limits of a 1-year funding period. The Pilot program structure includes the following 3 components:

1. Core Curriculum didactic blocks. A didactic Core is taught during 2 separate 3-week sessions through direct participation and problem-solving learning methods.
2. Attachment Site rotations. This phase consists of an experiential mentored assignment in which each fellow is attached to a host government agency, an NGO, or an academic institution to complete two 3-month assignments.
3. Posttraining program. The third phase provides virtual and in-person opportunities to continue to interact and collaborate with faculty, other fellowship graduates, and incoming fellows.

The proposed Fellowship is focused on African fellows, but it also includes some US fellows because it is thought that this mix will enhance the training experience for both groups of fellows. Furthermore, there is hope to create an international network of leaders that will be sustained long after completion of the Afya Bora Leadership Fellowship.

Pilot Program Structure

The structure of the Pilot program is summarized in **Table 2**.

Orientation

Before the first section of the Core Curriculum, a 2-day orientation is held for fellows and primary mentors. This orientation presents the overall goals of leadership training and the desired outcomes for fellows, mentors, faculty, and Afya Bora Consortium members. It describes expectations for Attachment Site rotations and explains the role of the primary mentor and the mentoring team. Orientation emphasizes effective mentoring and mentorship and the timeline for Attachment Site project reports. This session also stresses the importance of full participation by trainees, mentors, and Consortium members.

Core Curriculum Blocks

The Core Curriculum is taught at the African partner institutions and brings together the new cohort of 20 African and US trainees. The first 3-week segment is conducted at the University of Nairobi, Kenya and consists of three 1-week modules: (1) Leadership Skills, (2) Program and Project Management, and (3) Implementation Science and Health Systems Research. The second segment is conducted at the Muhimbili University of Health and Allied Sciences in Tanzania and consists of 3 additional 1-week modules: (4) Monitoring and Evaluation, (5) Technology and Bioinformatics, and (6) Communications and Media Skills. These topics are essential to global health leadership, yet they are rarely included in medical and nursing curricula.

Courses are taught by African and US instructors who collaborate to develop training materials, make presentations, and lead discussions. A variety of teaching methods are used, including problem-based learning in small groups and face-to-face didactics, supplemented, in some instances, by videotaped lectures and other distance learning resources. All modules highlight gaps in health care delivery and disease prevention and emphasize the research and policy priorities that are most relevant at the national and regional levels.

Table 2
Structure and timeline for the Pilot fellowship

Core Curriculum: 3 wk	Rotation: 3 mo	Core Curriculum: 3 wk	Rotation: 3 mo
2-d orientation	Independent projects at Attachment Sites	1-d project presentation	Independent projects at Attachment Sites
Core Curriculum: three 1-wk modules Leadership Program management Implementation science	1-d workshop for mentoring teams within the first 2 wk Weekly meetings with the primary mentor Semi-monthly meetings with the country lead and in-country fellows Monthly meetings with the mentoring team Project report due last day of rotation	Core Curriculum: three 1-wk modules Monitoring and evaluation Technology and bioinformatics Communications and media skills	1-d workshop for mentoring teams within the first 2 wk Weekly meetings with the primary mentor Semi-monthly meetings with the country lead and in-country fellows Monthly meetings with the mentoring team Project report due last day of rotation

The Core Curriculum modules are also available for in-service training. There are employed African health professionals who would like to take short courses to build their skills and increase their career opportunities. However, many of these health professionals cannot be released for a full 1- or 2-year fellowship. To respond to this need, the Pilot Program includes 4 places for trainees who will only take the Core Curriculum modules. If successful, this aspect of the program will be expanded in the future.

Attachment Site Rotations

Attachment Site is the term coined for organizations that operate in the African partner countries. Entities with the potential to serve as Attachment Sites include Ministries of Health, NGOs, PEPFAR missions, Centers for Disease Control and Prevention (CDC) field stations, USAIDS missions or offices, WHO regional offices or sites, and universities. Because AIDS is at present such a cross-cutting salient problem in the African partner countries, all the training projects involve human immunodeficiency virus (HIV)/AIDS issues. Working Group members visited more than 25 potential Attachment Sites between January and March 2010 in Botswana, Kenya, Tanzania, and Uganda and met with directors and senior staff who were uniformly enthusiastic about participating in the Afya Bora Fellowship.

A 3-month Attachment Site rotation takes place after each of the Core Curriculum blocks. During these rotations, fellows conduct independent projects. Potential areas of focus include clinical research, public health and disease prevention, health policy formulation, health systems research, implementation science, and program management and evaluation. All projects include some type of applied research experience.

A final report, which varies in length and format depending on the type of project and needs of the Attachment Site, is required at the end of each rotation.

The overarching goal is to prepare fellows to assume leadership roles in a variety of large-scale health programs, whether they are focused on specific diseases or on strengthening health systems. This experiential training provides fellows with skills that are relevant to effective leadership in many health areas so that they will have the flexibility to respond to evolving health needs of their countries.

During their time at their Attachment Sites, fellows are also encouraged to take occasional short courses, attend scientific meetings, and engage in skill-building activities that will support their career goals and job aspirations. Weekly meetings for fellows with their primary mentor are mandatory to discuss progress and review challenges. In each African partner country, a member of the Consortium Working Group serves as the country program leader. The program leader meets monthly with fellows in that country. This provides a forum for fellows to present their work and obtain input as they come together to review their projects, share experiences, and receive mentorship and group instruction. These meetings also help the trainees bond and form professional networks across Africa.

Fellow Recruitment and Selection

African fellows

For the Pilot program, the African partners advertise widely at all the in-country health centers and within their own Fellowship programs for health professionals interested in the program. Attachment Sites also have the opportunity to nominate their professional staff for the Pilot program. The aim is to select 12 African applicants to complete the Pilot Fellowship, 3 from each African partner country, with at least 1 professional in nursing or public health. As indicated earlier, an additional 4 African applicants are enrolled only in the Core Curriculum blocks.

There are challenges inherent in identifying "potential future global health leaders," and selecting the most promising fellows to maximize success of the fellowship is also important. A major criterion for selection is the commitment of candidates to work in-country health centers for 2 years after completion of the Pilot program, and this is assessed during the interview. In addition, the selection process seeks to optimize the gender balance among the trainees from each profession. The Consortium is committed to recruiting qualified graduate nurses to ensure a balance of trainees from different health professions. The schools of nursing at the African institutions are particularly enthusiastic about the Afya Bora Fellowship and make a major effort to identify appropriate candidates for the program.

The recruitment process begins with a written application form and letters of reference. Selected applicants are brought in for an interview with the Selection Committee. The Selection Committee is composed of 3 members of the Working Group, 3 representatives of potential Attachment Sites, and 1 or 2 members from collaborating academic health centers. The Committee seeks evidence of prior leadership activities and characteristics such as initiative, creativity, and strong interpersonal skills. Once the candidates are selected, there is a subsequent matching process in which trainees are interviewed by representatives of Attachment Sites and then ranked to optimize alignment between the objectives and interests of fellows and Attachment Sites.

US fellows

For the Pilot program, a total of 4 US trainees are accepted. The goal is to recruit individuals who will not only benefit greatly from the experience but also contribute unique perspectives and different approaches that will enhance the learning experience for all. Among the 4 US institutions, we will search for physicians and nurses who are already enrolled in post-doctoral fellowships or doctoral or master's programs and who have demonstrated a strong interest in global health. The US Consortium members have access to potential recruits through existing fellowship programs and those working in several specialties, such as adult and pediatric infectious diseases. The application process and selection of US fellows is otherwise similar to that described earlier for African fellows.

Mentoring

The success of experiential work at the Attachment Sites critically depends on supervision of each trainee by a primary mentor and a mentoring team. The mentoring team works with the primary mentor and fellow to select and develop the project and determines the skills and collaborations needed to complete it within the available time. Mentors are selected from the Attachment Sites to which trainees have been assigned and from the Consortium institutions. They include both African mentors who can provide on-site support and US mentors chosen for their expertise relevant to the activities of the trainees. The mentoring team is chosen considering the career interests of each fellow, a history of successful mentorship, and the nature of the project. Ideally, the primary mentor is identified before beginning the first Core Curriculum block. To emphasize the importance of this activity and maximize their active participation, African mentors are paid for their time.

All African mentors attend a 1-day mentoring workshop, which is held within 2 weeks before the Attachment Site rotation start date. US mentors are asked to attend selected portions via teleconference. During the first part of the workshop, mentors are given an intensive briefing regarding the goals of the program and their responsibilities. They are given a Mentoring Manual that sets forth established mentoring guidelines. This Manual was developed and refined at mentoring workshops that were held between April and September 2010 in Kenya, Botswana, Tanzania, and Uganda.

Program Evaluation

A formal monitoring and evaluation plan is tested during the Pilot program. For this purpose, the consortium is collaborating with the International Training and Education Center for Health (I-TECH). I-TECH is a collaborative center operated jointly by the University of Washington and the University of California in San Francisco. I-TECH has established a global network for building health care delivery capacity and training a skilled health workforce and has extensive experience in program evaluation. I-TECH has been commissioned to conduct an internal assessment using data they collect from faculty, mentors, Attachment Site staff, and fellows. The I-TECH evaluation includes an I-TECH observer who attends the Core Curriculum modules and may visit some of the Attachment Sites. I-TECH personnel collect and compile data throughout the Pilot program and prepare a summary for the wrap-up meeting to be conducted at the completion of the program.

As part of the internal assessment, trainees are evaluated for their achievement of competencies that are needed to operate effectively in domains such as leadership and management, health systems management, health service delivery, program evaluation, communications, bioinformatics, and research. Faculty, Attachment Site staff, and mentors are also asked to assess the performance of each fellow after each 3-week Core Curriculum block and Attachment Site rotation.

At the conclusion of the Pilot program, there is a wrap-up meeting of fellows, key faculty, Attachment Site staff, and mentors. This meeting evaluates the Pilot program by identifying its strengths, and weaknesses and recommending approaches for improvement. During the meeting, I-TECH conducts an anonymous evaluation by fellows of instructors, mentors, faculty, and Attachment Sites.

As part of the wrap-up meeting, a group of experts is convened to conduct an external assessment. The external assessment committee includes experts in program evaluation as well as African health leaders who have had experience with fellowship programs. The external assessment uses data collected by I-TECH and summarized in their preliminary report.

Roles and Responsibilities of African and US Partners

For the Afya Bora Consortium to be successful, it is essential to define the responsibilities and rewards for both the African and US partner institutions. The African partner institutions are putting their reputations and support behind the vision of the Consortium to provide a novel type of training for future health leaders in their countries. In addition, they are committing faculty effort, recruitment of outstanding trainees, and institutional resources to the program. The participating African faculty has contributed critical thinking to developing the vision for the Fellowship, with a combination of innovative ideas and reality testing, to ensure a culturally appropriate plan for the Fellowship. Potential rewards include access to external funding, an expanded role for their academic health training institutions, and a training opportunity that may help counter the brain drain problem.

The US institutions have contributed to the Afya Bora Consortium in several critical areas. They have provided some of the concepts that have inspired the Consortium vision, enthusiastic participation of global health faculty, and funding opportunities. The US institutions bring access to a wide array of schools in their Universities, including expertise in program development and management, monitoring, evaluating, and research technologies, both in health and nonhealth fields. The Afya Bora Consortium provides the US institutions with an important new opportunity to expand their global health programs and a robust global network that offers many resources for service, training, and research.

CONCLUDING COMMENTS

It is thought that the proposed Afya Bora Leadership Fellowship is an innovative model, which has several features that distinguish it from other existing fellowship programs, including:

- An African-centric focus emphasizing HIV/AIDS. Most trainees, training sites, faculty, and mentors are African or located in African partner countries. Training in research relevant to HIV/AIDS provides skills that can be used to address the current AIDS pandemic in Africa and serves as an entry point for addressing other health challenges in developing countries.
- Emphasis on leadership, evaluation skills, and practical experience to prepare trainees to lead large, evidence-based health programs. The model provides an integrated program to fill a critical health leadership gap that currently exists in many African nations, including the 4 African partner countries. It delivers leadership training and management skills to a select group of African and US health professionals early in their careers. Trainees are prepared to design, implement, evaluate, and iteratively improve large-scale programs that link research, preventive and curative health services, training, and policy development.

- Links to future employment. To proactively address the problem of brain drain among this talented pool of future leaders, the Fellowship emphasizes experiential learning assignments to in-country Attachment Sites during which trainees would conduct projects at organizations or agencies that could provide future employment, which is coupled with the clear responsibility of Mentoring Committees to facilitate posttraining placements. The commitment of African trainees is reinforced by a written agreement to work at in-country health centers for at least 2 years after completion of the program.
- The power of a Consortium. As stated earlier, the Consortium involves 8 academic health training institutions, each of which has a medical school, a nursing school, and (in many instances) a school of public health. In aggregate, the different partners bring a broad array of resources and opportunities to the Consortium, much more than any single twinning partnership. The involvement of multiple institutions greatly strengthens the fellowship program and increases its sustainability.
- Interdisciplinary framework across medicine, nursing, and other health-related disciplines. It is believed that training across disciplinary, geocultural, and gender lines is critical to the development of effective health leadership in Africa and around the globe. Therefore, integrating trainees from medicine, nursing, public health, and other relevant disciplines from the 5 participating countries to learn and work together is a crucial component of the program. The emphasis on nursing also helps advance interdisciplinary training and collaboration as well as achieve gender equity.
- Targeting sustainable African training capacity, not just trainees. A key long-term goal is to establish the training capacity of African institutions rather than just launching one more program to provide additional trainees. The eventual goal is to move the primary direction of this training program to the African partner institutions. The fellowship program is viewed as a catalyst for institutional development in research, education, clinical practice, and policy development. To this end, most of the training takes place in the African partner countries. The South-South partnership will play a major role in establishing a sustainable training program led by African institutions.
- Experiential training for US trainees in African programs. Another long-term goal of the program is to establish the capacity of US institutions to train US trainees in real-life programs of global health relevance. There is a cadre of junior US health professionals with a career interest in global health, which strongly desires immersion experiences in African health programs. Furthermore, training in a cohort with their African peers markedly enhances the impact of their international experiences. It offers emerging African and US global health leaders opportunities to develop critical thinking skills in cross-cultural negotiation and collaboration and launch the next generation of sustainable North-South and South-South partnerships.

Significance

During the frequent meetings and conference calls, it has become clear that the Afya Bora Consortium has enthusiastic support from the African partner institutions, which has endowed the proposal with significant credibility. In addition, the participation of a large number of African and US institutions markedly increases the probability that the program can be sustained on a long-term basis. The proposed Fellowship, once evaluated and refined, could be scaled up in several ways, such as (1) expanding the program by including other interested academic institutions in Africa and the United States, (2) replicating the program by initiating similar consortia, perhaps in other geographic areas, (3) using specific components of the program for in-service training of health service professionals in established positions or for strengthening existing training programs, and (4) including opportunities for fellows to do rotations outside Africa at international organizations, such as WHO, CDC, and UNAIDS. Thus, this model has the potential to have an impact that reaches beyond the immediate scope of the present Consortium, both in Africa and in the northern countries.[8–10]

ACKNOWLEDGMENTS

The Working Group of the Afya Bora Consortium includes Robert Bollinger, Carey Farquhar, Nancy Glass, Ephata Kaaya, James Kiarie, Yohana Mashalla, Gorrette Nalwadda, Marjorie Muecke, Neal Nathanson, Oathokwa Nkomazana, Teresa Odero, Thomas Quinn, Esther Seloilwe, Christopher Stewart, Nelson Sewankambo, Gloria Tshweneagaeg, Joachim Voss, and Judith Wasserheit. Their mailing addresses and e-mail addresses are provided in Appendix 1.

APPENDIX 1: MAILING AND E-MAIL ADDRESSES

Name	E-mail	Address
Robert Bollinger	rcb@jhmi.edu	Johns Hopkins Medical Institutions, 600 North Wolfe Street, Phipps 540, Baltimore, MD 21287, USA
Carey Farquhar	cfarq@u.washington.edu	International AIDS Research and Training Program, Departments of Medicine, Epidemiology, and Global Health, University of Washington, 325 Ninth Avenue, Box 359909, Seattle, WA 98104, USA
Nancy Glass	nglass1@son.jhmi.edu	Johns Hopkins University School of Nursing, 525 North Wolfe Street, Room 439, Baltimore, MD 21205-2110, USA
Ephata Kaaya	ekaaya@muhas.ac.tz	Muhimbili University of Health and Allied Sciences, PO Box 65001, Dar es Salaam, Tanzania
James Kiarie	jkiarie@swiftkenya.com	University of Nairobi, College of Health Sciences, Department of Obstetrics and Gynecology, PO Box 19767-00202, Nairobi 00202, Kenya
Yohana Mashalla	yohana.mashalla@mopipi.ub.bw	School of Medicine, University of Botswana, Kgogolamoko House, Private Bag 00713 Gaborone, Botswana

(*continued on next page*)

APPENDIX 1 *(continued)*

Name	E-mail	Address
Gorette Nalwadda	gnalwadda@gmail.com	Department of Nursing, School of Health Sciences, Makerere University, PO Box 7072, Kampala 256, Uganda
Marjorie Muecke	muecke@nursing.upenn.edu	School of Nursing, University of Pennsylvania, 257 Fagin Hall, Philadelphia, PA 19104 6020, USA
Neal Nathanson	nathansn@upenn.edu	Global Health Programs, 1007 Blockley Hall, School of Medicine, University of Pennsylvania, Philadelphia, PA 19104-6021, USA
Oathokwa Nkomazana	Oathokwa2000@yahoo.com	School of Medicine, University of Botswana, PO Box 40670, Gaborone, Botswana
Teresa Odero	Oderoteresa@yahoo.com	University of Nairobi, School of Nursing, Box 30197-00100, Nairobi, Kenya
Thomas Quinn	tquinn2@jhmi.edu	Johns Hopkins University School of Medicine, Hampton House 180, 624 North Broadway, Baltimore, MD 21205, USA
Esther Seloilwe	SELOILWE@mopipi.ub.bw	School of Nursing, University of Botswana, Private Bag 0022, Gaborone, Botswana
Christopher Stewart	CStewart@sfghpeds.ucsf.edu	University of California San Francisco Box SFGH, MS 6E/SFGH (nh) San Francisco, CA 94143–SFGH, USA
Nelson Sewankambo	sewankam@infocom.co.ug	College of Health Sciences, Makerere University, Kampala 7072, Uganda
Gloria Tshweneagae	tshweneagaeg@mopipi.ub.bw	University of Botswana School of Nursing, Private Bag 0022, Gaborone, Botswana
Joachim Voss	vossj@u.washington.edu	School of Nursing, University of Washington, Box 357266, Seattle, WA 98195-7266, USA
Judith Wasserheit	jwasserh@uw.edu	Department of Global Health Schools of Medicine and Public Health, University of Washington, 325 Ninth Avenue, Seattle, WA 98109, USA

REFERENCES

1. Kameri-Mbote P. The operational environment and constraints for NGOs in Kenya: strategies for good policy and practice. IELRC Working Paper 2000-2, published by The International Environmental Law Research Institute, Geneva (Switzerland). Available at: http://www.ielrc.org/content/w0002.pdf. Accessed February 12, 2011.
2. Accordia Global Health Foundation. Building healthcare leadership in Africa: a call to action. Washington, DC: Accordia Global Health Foundation; 2009.
3. Accordia Global Health Foundation. Return on investment: the long-term impact of building health care capacity in Africa. Washington, DC: Accordia Global Health Foundation; 2010.

4. Global Health Council. Developing health leadership through the global health initiative: a proposal from the health systems roundtable of the global health council. Washington, DC: Global Health Council; 2009.
5. Quinn TC. The Johns Hopkins center for global health: transcending borders for world health. Acad Med 2008;83:134–42.
6. Macfarlane SB, Agabian N, Novotny TE, et al. Think globally, act locally, and collaborate internationally: global health sciences at the University of California, San Francisco. Acad Med 2008;83:173–9.
7. Kanter SL. Global health is more important in a smaller world. Acad Med 2008;83: 115–6.
8. Macfarlane SB, Jacobs M, Kaaya EE. In the name of global health: trends in academic institutions. J Public Health Policy 2008;29:383–401.
9. Hotez PJ. Training the next generation of global health scientists: a school of appropriate technology for global health. PLoS Negl Trop Dis 2008;2:e279, 1–4.
10. Drain PK, Holmes KK, Skeff KM, et al. Global health training and international clinical rotations during residency: current status, needs, and opportunities. Acad Med 2009;84:320–5.

Medical Education: Meeting the Challenge of Implementing Primary Health Care in Sub-Saharan Africa

Mushtaq Ahmed, MBBS, FRCS[a,*], Camer W. Vellani, MD, FRCP[b], Alex O. Awiti, PhD[c]

KEYWORDS

• Medical education • Primary health care • Sub-Saharan Africa

The ideas expressed in this discourse have been derived from the experience of planning for undergraduate medical education at the Aga Khan University (AKU) Medical College, Nairobi, which is a private university for the East African region; broad-based general education and the principles of liberal arts are incorporated in the curriculum.

Medical education in sub-Saharan Africa (SSA) must be defined by its health needs and the health care services required. This article begins by describing the sociodemographic milieu that determines the disease pattern. Then it considers the compelling case for primary health care (PHC) in the context of community participation and multisector development as the driver of a medical education plan. An attempt is made to define the attributes of a doctor required to be effective in the region and to anticipate the inevitable challenges that lie ahead, including authorization and implementation of the plan as well as productive retention of graduates in the region, their professional development, and their contributions to the efficiency of health care. The potential roles of the AKU and the wider Aga Khan Development Network (AKDN) in East Africa are discussed in this regard.

THE HEALTH CONTEXT

The population in SSA is largely rural. Access to health care is difficult in the absence of good roads and transport. Rural people are mostly subsistence farmers,

---

The authors have nothing to disclose.
[a] The Aga Khan University Medical College, 3rd Parklands Avenue, PO Box 30270, 00100, Nairobi, Kenya
[b] The Aga Khan University, Stadium Road, PO Box 3500, Karachi 74800, Pakistan
[c] The Aga Khan University, 3rd Parklands Avenue, PO Box 30270, 00100, Nairobi, Kenya
* Corresponding author.
E-mail address: mushtaq.ahmed@aku.edu

doi:10.1016/j.idc.2011.02.011

pastoralists, and fisherman, whose livelihood depends on natural resources. A high dependence on the climate for food security without adequate capacity to adapt to climate change has consequences for nutrition and health.[1] As the fastest growing region of the world (annual growth rate 2.4%) the population of SSA, currently at 840 million, is expected to double in just 30 years.[2] Half the population is younger than 18 years[2]; as it grows older the incidence of chronic disease will increase. Urbanization is gaining momentum, and by 2050 it is expected that 67% of the population in SSA, 1 billion people, will reside in towns and cities.[3] In urban areas there are unplanned settlements of migrant populations, such as Kibera in Nairobi where nearly 0.5 million people live in unhygienic conditions. Moreover, urbanization exposes inhabitants to unhealthy lifestyles that predispose to chronic disease. Desperate economic situations lead to increased crime and violence, with its attendant consequences for health and social harmony. More than 40% of people in SSA are extremely poor, earning less than US$1 a day, and 30% moderately so, earning between US$1 and US$2.[4] For various reasons it seems that the intended halving of extreme poverty by 2015 will not be achieved and that poverty in one form or another will continue to be a major determinant of ill health. Poverty leads not only to material deprivation and lack of access to basic services but also disempowerment due to lack of autonomy and freedom of expression.[5] The predilection of women in their reproductive years to human immunodeficiency virus (HIV)-AIDS in SSA exemplifies the consequences of these conditions. By inference from indicators of good health in relatively poor countries like Sri Lanka, Mechanic[6] suggests that education, empowerment of women, and the provision of basic health services have independent roles in determining health status. From a population health perspective, the impact of poverty on early child development is particularly distressing; adversities during intrauterine life and early childhood are biologically embedded and lead to cognitive impairment, behavioral disorders, developmental delay, and health impairments in later life.[7,8] Of course, poor health itself predisposes to social deprivation; hence, alleviation of poverty is dependent on addressing the health-related Millennium Development Goals (MDGs).

As a consequence of the interplay between social, demographic, and environmental factors, communicable and noncommunicable diseases (NCD) coexist in SSA.[9] NCD and effectively controlled HIV-AIDS comprise an increasing burden of chronic disease[10] requiring not only long-term health care but concurrently the maintenance of useful lives through employment, such that the economic welfare of the family and normal child development are assured. A PHC approach could be adopted to keep patients with chronic disease out of hospital for as long as they remain stable.

Maternal and neonatal mortality rates continue to be unacceptably high in SSA.[11] Although mortality in children younger than 5 years has improved worldwide, in SSA the decline in deaths, especially from malaria, has been less impressive.[9] PHC is well placed for the management of the bulk of problems related to maternal, neonatal, and child health (MNCH). Because PHC is situated in communities, it can be strengthened also to manage and refer other prevalent problems such as nutritional disorders, trauma, and mental illness, which require multidisciplinary or multisectoral interventions at district level.

THE CASE FOR PRIMARY HEALTH CARE

Having identified MNCH issues and chronic diseases as major health problems, and social and demographic factors including inequity in the distribution of health services as root causes, a logical approach to improving the health of the population might include: universal and equitable access to health care including health promotion, disease prevention, curative care, and rehabilitation; a comprehensive approach integrating PHC with community participation and multisector development; a reliance on trained community health workers (CHW) to deliver elements of health care to families and the community; accessible center-based health care for management of unstable clinical states; efficient systems for provision of drugs and equipment, health information, supervision, and training; and the selective referral of patients for specialist care.[12] In this regard, the district is the smallest organizational entity with managerial responsibility and some financial authority to improve the health of the population (100,000–500,000 in SSA districts) within a defined geographic area. The district is supported by national health strategies and policies.[13]

On the 30th anniversary of the Alma Ata declaration, its advocacy for PHC as a means of meeting the health-related MDGs was renewed. The experience of the last 30 years has shown a decline in the mortality rate in children younger than 5 years in 30 low-income and middle-income countries worldwide, with Thailand in the forefront, who have made progress with PHC and identified the following factors linked to success: national commitment; health systems integration; devolution to the district level; use of CHWs; and removal of financial barriers to an essential health package.[14]

Although success so far may be limited, emerging concepts in PHC make its prospects for the twenty-first century promising. Such factors include: technological innovations, for example, the use of mobile phones for tele-health; improved access as a result of trained health workers permeating homes, work places, and schools; innovative financial schemes for health; incentive-based human resource management; multisector development encompassing education, agriculture, infrastructure, and income generation; research-based evidence for best practices; the rights revolution with people demanding equity, high quality, and respect from health providers as well as protection from health hazards; and active engagement of the population in their health care as coproducers of health and as a source of funding.[15]

THE DOCTORS' ROLE IN SUPPORTING PHC

While acknowledging that PHC's success is dependent on teamwork, it is important to question the role of doctors. Failure to attract doctors has led to nonphysicians filling the void in many African district health services. As a rule, nonphysicians have lower secondary school achievements and receive only 3 to 4 years of clinical training of variable standard.[16] Although they may have useful roles, at present only the public is the arbiter of their performance. Their advantage is that they are more easily retained at lower pay in underserved communities to which many belong.[16] Although equipped for pattern recognition and simple algorithmic intervention, their basic knowledge of structure, function, and mechanisms of disease is insufficient to understand and rationally manage less familiar clinical presentations. It is clear that one of the doctor's roles should be to define and contribute to the professional training of other health care personnel. In addition, the doctor in the team must assess the needs and support for health care, appraise the effectiveness of the service, and search scientifically for evidence to aid understanding and management of diseases prevalent in the community, in collaboration with professionals who have the requisite expertise. When medical officers without a specialist qualification in family medicine are posted to district health services, they must perform better than nondoctor surrogates; however, without appropriate postgraduate education and training even they are not prepared for full utilization of their potential abilities. Family physicians especially trained for PHC, who can recognize and manage a range of diseases and are prepared to investigate their underlying root causes in the community, are the obvious first choice. Family medicine training has been going on in South Africa for 15 years and is presently accepted as an area of specialization, as it is also in Kenya and Rwanda.[17]

Shortage and maldistribution of doctors overall is, however, a major problem. There are on average 13 doctors per 100,000 people in SSA, compared with 164 in the United Kingdom and 274 in the United States, and they are mostly based in the cities.[18] The design of a PHC system clearly must optimize the engagement of doctors, who comprise the most expensive element in the system. Nonphysicians ostensibly can be trained to recognize and manage common clinical problems or follow a plan of management of more complex illness defined by the physician after one consultation, provided the physician receives feedback from the nondoctor attendant and is available for referral if something either unanticipated or unusual occurs. In Mexico, the doctor's role has been successfully optimized by using mobile phone technology to coordinate care.[19]

MEDICAL EDUCATION

Based on the preceding discussion, the practicing medical doctor in SSA should have acquired the attributes given here.

An Understanding of the Importance of the Social Determinants of Health and Illness

Chantler[20] wrote:

> *The main task for a doctor is diagnosis. Working out what is wrong and why it is wrong requires knowledge of biomedical and behavioral science and an understanding of people and the society in which they live. The purpose of education at university and medical school is to ensure this is achieved, and to provide a sound foundation for continued learning throughout a professional career.*

While this stated purpose of medical education may be self evident, in reality it is not the prevailing model of medical practice. Most medical practice is centered round the diagnosis of an illness and its immediate causative or risk factors. For example, doctors are not usually concerned about why individuals in an endemic zone for malaria are not protected against mosquito bites, or what determines the lifestyle and diets of patients with coronary artery disease. To remedy this problem, the objectives of medical education must be widened to include consideration of factors influencing human development through various stages of life, from a fetus to an adult, that also influence health. The factors include maternal education, nutrition and health before conception, normal gestation, safe birth and survival of mother and child, nutrition and nurturing, the social environment of the infant and child, access to competent health care, education from pre-primary to secondary school, technical and higher education, conditions of work, family beliefs and behavior, the influence of teachers, peers, and role models, as well as a host of other social, cultural, political, economic, and environmental conditions. Some of these factors may affect gene expression and consequently influence learning ability, health, and behavior of the individual and collectively the society, which in turn creates unfavorable conditions for early child development.[21] A sustainable, coordinated effort by multiple sectors of government, with civil society and communities, is necessary to improve human development indices and population health.

An Understanding of the Bio-Psychosocial Model of Care and Health Systems

In Africa, most doctors gravitate to large public or private hospitals in the cities and often deal with once controllable disease, now advanced with multiple comorbidities and complications. The prevalent model of hospital care ignores the origin of disease and factors conditioning its progression, such as geographic, financial, social, and cultural limitations of access to health care, compliance with treatment, ability to cope with illness, and continuity of care. Two conclusions emerge from this disconnection: (1) doctors need to understand the greater benefits of the bio-psychosocial model of health care, and (2) should contribute to developing a system of health care delivery that could avoid or ameliorate many of the clinical problems they deal with. The objectives of such a system should be to promote health, prevent disease, provide timely intervention, and refer patients selectively to higher levels of care, with concern for cost effectiveness.

On graduation and after completing a period of mandatory internship during which the doctor assumes direct responsibility for patients and works under close supervision, he or she should have the ability and the opportunity to develop further as a clinical specialist, a generalist, a population health practitioner, a scientist, or a manager. This pluripotency is an asset for an integrated pyramidal health care delivery system that is committed to the holistic concept of primary health care, and its provision for appropriate referral of complex problems.

Clinical Competence

Clinical competence of a high order distinguishes an effective medical doctor from other health professionals. The authors use the term clinical competence in a composite sense to include: (a) the basic skills of clinical observation, investigation, and reasoned diagnosis and management of illness based on knowledge concepts emanating from biologic and biomedical sciences; (b) empathy, a caring attitude, and ethical professional behavior; (c) practical skills of communication with patients and relatives, performing commonly required procedures, and managing emergencies; (d) interpersonal skills of communication and collaboration.

Effective communication with culturally diverse and socially disadvantaged people deserves special mention. The considerable cultural heterogeneity among Africans requires an understanding of how different beliefs and practices influence illness, and how differences across cultures influence attitudes to illness: for example, understanding who makes the decisions in the family, the role of women in decision making, belief in the notion that illness is due to fate, the importance given to spiritual and other forms of healing and religious taboos, and the ideations that exist about death and dying. The doctor should be able to exercise a nonjudgmental approach to community-specific norms of behavior, such as "bride price," which prevents women in certain African cultures from giving informed consent for interventional procedures,[22] and social stigmas attached to illness such as HIV infection. Evidence indicates that the ability of health services to deal effectively with diverse cultural and social conditions reduces inequity in health care and improves health outcomes.[23]

A major source of inefficiency and ineffectiveness of PHC is poor management of resources.[24] Health personnel need to be trained and motivated continually to do good work together as a team. Doctors trained as family physicians are well placed to provide training and supervision for health care and to appraise health workers' performance, as well as being well positioned to direct the cost-effective use of resources through coordination of evidence-based care.

CHALLENGES FOR EDUCATION

A significant factor to consider is that in SSA, entrants to medical college are 17- to 18-year-old high school leavers. Selection is highly competitive and based on academic achievement, placing potential candidates from underprivileged communities at a disadvantage. Evidence from South Africa indicates that students from rural areas are more likely to work after graduation in underserved areas.[25] Diversity of students' geographic, cultural, and socioeconomic backgrounds could also facilitate communication with patients, communities, and health services. However, ensuring a diverse student body is not easy. It will require enhancement of school education in underprivileged areas, assessment of students' competence to study medicine in English, and consideration of attributes besides academic achievement, as well as students' attitude toward social service and tolerance of diverse cultures. If promising candidates need improvement in English language proficiency, due to lack of opportunity, facilities to prepare them for higher education will be necessary. Financial subsidies will be required for students from economically underprivileged families for 6 years of education.

Expanding students' knowledge horizon to include understanding of human development and values of responsible citizenship requires broad-based general education. A 4-year North American style of liberal arts education could not be adopted as practiced; it requires time that competes with the opportunity cost of contributing to health care and earning a living, on the one hand, and adds significantly to the cost of education on the other. Nevertheless, the concept of acquiring broad-based knowledge, skills of reasoning, self-directed learning, problem solving, teamwork, communication, reflection on one's experience and beliefs, as well as tolerance of diversity of thought and culture is germane to the practice of medicine. Just how such a foundation can be provided and seamlessly melded into professional education without extending the period of study beyond 6 years requires imaginative curriculum planning, careful consideration of essential knowledge for professional practice in the context of the health service for which undergraduates are being prepared, and instructional strategies that enable efficient learning of concepts. A strong foundation of biomedical and population health sciences, as discussed earlier, is essential for solving clinical problems. Thoughtful faculty with experience in education and health sciences will be required; such individuals will be engaged in active, relevant research. This approach means that the medical school must provide appropriate support for laboratory-based and community-based research. These resources will also support graduate programs that should prepare the next generation of faculty.

Clinical and community-based experiences should begin early, preferably in the context of integrated PHC. Family medicine could provide the foundation for experience in PHC. It is essential for at least part of the experience to be gained in conditions of health care that are widely prevalent in SSA. For a private medical school this requires partnership with the public sector; sadly there are no relevant examples of public-private partnership to learn from. There are other problems too: facilities for training in family medicine are few at undergraduate and postgraduate levels, role models are scarce, and livelihood as a primary care physician in the community is threatened by competition from specialist clinicians on the one hand and nonphysician clinical officers and pharmacists on the other.

Selecting 17- and 18-year-olds to study medicine is a serious responsibility that should anticipate a "change of mind." Provisions should be made for alternative careers, otherwise attrition will ensue and intellectual talent will be wasted. A natural point of transition occurs after 4 years of study, before concentration on clinical science begins. At this juncture it would be appropriate to award a BA in Health Sciences. Students who do not wish to pursue clinical medicine and those wishing to digress for a spell of research could follow new paths creditably.

Finally, clinical competence should be gauged by aligning teaching-learning strategies and educational assessment to professional outcomes and making provision for experiential learning. The competence is finally put to test during the internship year, when the graduates have direct responsibility for patient care under supervision. Continuous monitoring of graduates in practice will be necessary to judge whether the curricular objectives are attained.

RECRUITMENT AND RETENTION OF MEDICAL GRADUATES IN THE HEALTH SERVICES OF SSA

Assuming that medical education is successful, will the health service engage the graduates productively? Significant gaps exist in integration of PHC with community participation and multisector development, as well as in referral systems to higher levels of health care. The functions of health services are affected by deficient governance, management, funding, training of personnel, equipment and medical supplies, information systems, and operational research to inform policy and planning. Without opportunities to contribute to change, graduates working in PHC services may not continue for long, especially if they are not able to sustain themselves financially when they have a family of their own to feed, clothe, and educate. Graduates from poor communities may continue in service for a longer period; however, they will be disillusioned if their effort is not supported adequately by government. Persistence of unsatisfactory conditions of work and limited opportunities for professional development will encourage migration of doctors, and insufficiency of professionals will be a recurrent problem.

THE POTENTIAL ROLE OF AKU AND AKDN

The AKDN is a group of private, international, nondenominational agencies in specific regions of the developing world with a wide range of mandates, for example, health, education, and rural development. The AKDN promotes private sector enterprise working closely with communities and governments to respond to cultural, economic, and social challenges on an ongoing basis. AKU is a component of AKDN.

AKU started with a Faculty of Health Sciences in Pakistan 25 years ago. It now has an international presence, with diverse programs in several countries. In East Africa it offers advanced nursing studies (ANS), postgraduate medical education (PGME), and graduate programs in educational development. It is being developed to become a comprehensive university for the region, with a Faculty of Arts and Sciences (FAS) in Arusha, Tanzania and a Faculty of Health Sciences (FHS) in Nairobi, Kenya, with a Medical College and a School of Nursing and Midwifery. The concurrent development of FAS and FHS provides significant opportunities. Students entering the University will receive broad-based general education during their first 2 years, irrespective of whether they intend to pursue studies in medicine, nursing, or a degree program in the social sciences, arts, humanities, natural sciences, or mathematics. In medicine, the university already provides PGME and plans to offer graduate studies leading to Master's degrees and PhDs. Doctors will be educated and trained to become family physicians, clinical generalists, specialists or subspecialists, population health practitioners, or biomedical scientists. Finally, under the overarching theme of social and economic determinants of health, there is likely to be significant interdisciplinary research collaboration between FHS, FAS, and other international programs of the university.

In East Africa an integrated AKDN health care system is being planned that will incorporate the AKDN health services in the region and involve partnerships with service providers in the public and nongovernmental organization sectors. Partnership at the level of the district health services in the public sector is likely to be particularly rewarding, as it involves raising the standard of care in that sector. In the Coast Province of Kenya the Aga Khan Foundation has been promoting early childhood development and preschool education, water and sanitation programs, agricultural yield, and income generation. The Community Health Department of the Aga Khan Health Service, working with the government, has developed a Health Management Information System and is training health workers at the community and facilities levels, as well as providing courses of study in health systems management. In addition the ANS program has been upgrading the knowledge and skills of nurses who are in service in the public and private sectors. AKU's training programs in family medicine, nursing, and midwifery, and its research programs centered round the social and economic determinants of health could potentially provide the much-needed impetus for developing an integrated PHC model in collaboration with other AKDN agencies, the government, and international universities interested in global health. This approach could form a model of health care supported by appropriate education and training that might encourage retention of doctors and stimulate integration of social services for health care in other parts of SSA.

SUMMARY

Basic considerations of a conceptual plan for undergraduate medical education at the AKU Medical College, Nairobi, designed for graduates to function effectively in PHC in the public sector, are presented.

The plan responds to the adverse social, economic, environmental, and demographic factors that will continue to play a major part in determining the disease burden in SSA and the suitability of PHC to address health problems emanating from this situation. The crucial role of doctors specially trained in family medicine to support PHC is emphasized. Their roles could be optimized if they trained other health personnel to manage routine problems and follow instructions for continuity of care of more complex problems, asking for review of their work in an appropriate and timely manner. A doctor's clinical competence underpinned by sound scientific concepts and supported by principles of management is highly desirable for establishing functional links with the community and government sectors involved in human and community development.

However, the functions and sustainability of PHC require significant planning and development in partnership with government. Of crucial importance are requirements for development of faculty, education and training of health service personnel including those involved in health service management, research to support education and service, and development and sustenance of an effective health service.

It is proposed that AKU has the necessary potential in terms of the breadth and depth of its educational programs, its research focus on the social determinants of health, its immersion in communities and partnership with government as part of the wider AKDN, and its collaborative relationship with international organizations interested in global health to develop a model of medical education for the East African region that is supportive of primary health care.

REFERENCES

1. Development and Climate Change. The World Bank Group at work—a progress report 2008. Available at: www.worldbank.org/climate. Accessed October 9, 2010.

2. Ringheim K, Gribble J. Improving the reproductive health of sub Saharan Africa's youth: a route to achieve the millennium development goals. Washington, DC: Population Reference Bureau; 2010. popref@prb.org.
3. Goldstone J. The new population bomb: the four megatrends that will change the world. Foreign Aff 2010. p. 31–43.
4. Sachs JD. The end of poverty. New York: Penguin Press; 2005. p. 22–3.
5. Marmot M, Friel S, Beel R, et al. Closing the gap in a generation: health equity through action on the social determinants of health. Lancet 2008;372:1161–9.
6. Mechanic D. Population health: challenges for science and society. Milibank Q 2007;85:533–59.
7. Shonkoff JP, Boyce WT, McEwen BC. Neuroscience, molecular biology, and the childhood roots of health disparities: building a new framework for health promotion and disease prevention. JAMA 2009;301:2252–9.
8. Mustard JF. Early child development and experience-based brain development: scientific underpinnings of the importance of early child development in a globalized world. In: Young ME, editor. Early child development: from measurement to action—a priority for growth and equity. Washington, DC: The World Bank; 2007. p. 43–86.
9. Lopez AD, Mathers CD, Ezzati M, et al. Global and regional burden of disease and risk factors, 2001: systemic analysis of population health data. Lancet 2006;367:1747–51.
10. Tollman SM, Kahn K, Sartorius B, et al. Implications of mortality transition for primary health care in rural South Africa; a population-based surveillance study. Lancet 2008;372:893–901.
11. Bhutta ZA, Chopra M, Axelson H, et al. Countdown to 2015 decade report (2000-10): taking stock of maternal, newborn, and child survival. Lancet 2010;375: 2032–44.
12. Lawn JE, Rohde J, Rifkin S, et al. Alma Ata: rebirth and revision 1. Alma Ata 30 years on: revolutionary, relevant, and time to revitalise. Lancet 2008;372:917–27.
13. Eckman B, Pathmanathan I, Liljestarnd J. Alma Ata: rebirth and revision 7. Integrating health interventions for women, newborn babies, and children: a framework for action. Lancet 2008;372:990–1000.
14. Rohde J, Cousens S, Chopra M, et al. Alma Ata: rebirth and revision 4. 30 years after Alma Ata has primary care worked in countries? Lancet 2008;372:950–61.
15. Fenk J. Reinventing primary health care: the need for systems integration. Lancet 2009;374:170–3.
16. Mullan F, Frehywot S. Non-physician clinicians in 47 sub-Saharan African countries. Lancet 2007;370:2158–63.
17. De Maeseneer J, Flinkenflogel M. Primary health care in Africa: do family physicians fit in? Br J Gen Pract 2010;60:286–92.
18. Hagopian A, Thompson MJ, Fordyce M, et al. The migration of physicians from sub-Saharan Africa to the United States of America: measures of the African brain drain. Hum Resour Health 2004;2:17.
19. Knapp T, Richardson B, Viranna S. Three practical steps to better health for Africa: a new model to make care more accessible to Africa's people is not only possible but affordable. McKinsey Quarterly 2010. p. 1–8.
20. Chantler C. The role and education of doctors in the delivery of health care. Lancet 1999;353:950–61.
21. Early Child Development. A powerful equalizer. In: Irwin LG, Siddiqi A, Hertzman C, editors. Final report for the WHOs commission on social determinants of health. Available at: http://whqlibdoc.who.int/hq/2007/a91213.pdf. Accessed October 9, 2010.

22. Irabor D, Omonzejele P. Local attitudes, moral obligation, customary obedience and other cultural practices: their influence on the process of gaining informed consent for surgery in a tertiary institution in a developing country. Dev World Bioeth 2009;9:34–42.
23. Tervalon M. Components of culture in health for medical students' education. Acad Med 2003;78:570–6.
24. Coovadia H, Jewkes R, Barron P, et al. The health and health system of South Africa: historical roots of current public health challenges. Lancet 2009;374:817–34.
25. Tumbo JM, Couper ID, Hugo JFM. Rural origin of health science students at South African universities. S Afr Med J 2009;99:54–6.

Health of Migrants: Working Towards a Better Future

Xochitl Castañeda, MA[a,*], Magdalena Ruiz Ruelas, MPH[a], Emily Felt, MPP[a], Marc Schenker, MD, MPH[b]

KEYWORDS

- Mexican immigrants • Migration • Latino health
- Health insurance

In a world where profound inequalities exist, migration continues to be a fact of life. While migration enhances the diversity of nations, it also brings about a number of challenges, in particular when addressing health and social welfare. Countries are faced with the challenge of not only understanding and acknowledging the specific needs of migrant populations, but most importantly of finding the best way to meet those needs in the context of social, economic, and political pressures.

Regardless of the individual motivations behind migration, the experience presents a series of health challenges. For international migrants, in particular for those who cross without the required documentation, there are a number of health threats and problems that may begin during transit. These include contracting disease, becoming sick en route, and a series of physical and emotional effects caused by moving across borders that may be dangerous and with increased propensity for violence. It is important to note, however, that migration, in and of itself, does not exclusively lead to poor health; it is the stress of the migration process and the inequities that migrants face in their host country that exacerbates the risks to health and threatens their livelihood. Governments face the challenge of integrating the health needs of migrants into national plans, policies, and strategies, taking into account the human rights of these individuals, including their right to health. Not doing so creates marginalized groups in society, infringement on migrants' rights, and poor public health practice.[1] On the other hand, health professionals need to understand why people migrate, the situations they live in, and the factors influencing their health-seeking behaviors.

The authors have nothing to disclose.
[a] Health Initiative of the Americas, University of California at Berkeley, School of Public Health, 1950 Addison Street, Suite 203, Berkeley, CA 94704, USA
[b] Migration and Health Research Center, University of California Davis School of Medicine, MS1-C, One Shields Avenue, University of California at Davis, Davis, CA 95616, USA
* Corresponding author.
E-mail address: xochitl.castaneda@berkeley.edu

Infect Dis Clin N Am 25 (2011) 421–433
doi:10.1016/j.idc.2011.02.008 id.theclinics.com
0891-5520/11/$ – see front matter

There have been many articles focused on infectious and chronic diseases among migrants,[2–4] but few tackle the social determinants of health in this population. The authors will approach this article from that perspective in presenting the health status of Mexican immigrants in the United States. They first discuss access to health care and then look at the social determinants of health among this population and its impact on the health of Mexican immigrants, with a focus on women and children.

The article looks at Mexican immigrants, because they are the largest and fastest growing immigrant group in the United States, and they are likely to remain so for the foreseeable future. It is estimated that one-third of all foreign-born people and two-thirds of all foreign-born Latinos in the United States are from Mexico. As a prominent group in the United States, the health of this community is a concern for all Americans today and for future generations. While the length of this article does not allow for an extensive look at the health status of Mexican immigrants in the United States, the authors hope the overview provided will increase awareness among clinical practitioners of some of the specific health issues affecting this population and will help create better solutions to health concerns of this vulnerable population.

METHODS

Much of the data presented in this article come from the annual Migration and Health Issues Reports produced through joint efforts between the National Population Council of Mexico (CONAPO by its Spanish acronym) and the Health Initiative of the Americas (HIA) at the University of California Berkeley School of Public Health in collaboration with the University of California Migration and Health Research Center (MAHRC) at the University of California Davis. For the past 6 years, these organizations have collaborated to publish annual Health Issues Reports as part of a Migration and Health report series that details current demographic trends in the health of Latino immigrant groups in the United States. Specifically, the series has dedicated full reports to the US populations of Mexican, Central American, Colombian, and Ecuadorian descent in the United States. Issues have been devoted to health access and health insurance matters, and other significant health issues among Latinos in the United States. Demographic data for these reports are based on estimates from CONAPO derived from the US Department of the Census' Current Population Survey and the National Health Interview Survey.

For this article, information was drawn from the annual health issues reports on Immigration, Health and Work: The Facts behind the Myths[5]; Latinos in the United States[6]; The Children of Mexican Immigrants in the U.S.[7]; and Mexican Immigrant Women in the U.S.[8] Information was updated with other relevant sources including, demographic data from the US Department of the Census and other relevant immigrant health. Data on occupational health also were gathered from the Bureau of Labor Statistics, as were data from the US Department of Health and Human Services.

RESULTS

While the last 4 decades have seen a prominent shift and increase in migration, human movement is not a new phenomenon. Whether stemming from international forces or domestic migration as a result of rural-to-urban relocation, the movement of people is one of the driving forces for the formation of the modern world. Currently, over 214 million people worldwide live outside of their home country.[9]

The United States: A Nation of Immigrants

In the United States, immigration has been a major source of population growth and cultural change throughout much of the country's history, and it can be argued the entire US population (minus Native Americans) originated as immigrants. Today and throughout its history, the United States has been one of the most prominent receiving countries for international migration. The country is currently home to over 38 million (US Census) or 42 million immigrants (according to the IOM), comprising approximately 12% of the total US population. Of those 38 million immigrants, 53.6% were born in Latin America.[10] This included an estimated 12 million undocumented immigrants, of whom 56%—6.7 million people—were born in Mexico, followed by El Salvador, Guatemala, and Honduras.[11] Several other Latin American countries figure among the top 10 sources of undocumented immigration, including Brazil and Ecuador.[12] The Latino population is one of the fastest growing groups in the United States, and it is estimated that by 2050, Latinos will comprise about 25% of the total population.[13]

Mexican Immigrants in the United States—An Overview

According to the Census Bureau's American Community Survey, a total of 30.7 million Latinos of Mexican origin resided in the United States in 2008, making them the largest immigrant group in the country.[14] Nearly 4 in 10 (37.0%) reported being born in Mexico.[14] The Mexican origin population in the United State is younger than the US population and Latinos overall; the median age of Mexican immigrants is 25, while the median ages of the US population and all Latinos are 36 and 27, respectively.[14]

Despite being the largest immigrant group in the United States, Mexicans are one of the most disadvantaged populations in terms of education, earnings, and legal residence status. In 2007, 58% of non-elderly Mexican adults in the United States did not have a high-school degree, and it is estimated that 60% of all Mexican immigrants, and 80% to 85% of recent Mexican immigrants, are undocumented.

While there undoubtedly exist cultural, social, and family ties that surround the migration processes taking place between Mexico and the United States, the role that Mexicans so prominently display in the US workforce is a clear indicator of their primary motivation for migrating. Mexican recent immigrant men have a workforce participation rate of nearly 94% in the United States.[15] In comparison, there is a substantially smaller proportion of US-born, non-Latino white men participating in the workforce (84.8%).

The distribution of the Mexican immigrant population in the labor market is paradoxically associated with their poor access to health care services and health insurance. Whereas normally employment is associated with increased health care benefits, the opposite is the case with Mexican immigrants. In fact, their disadvantages in terms of health insurance are associated with the demand for labor that stimulates migration and places immigrants into poorly paid, often-dangerous jobs that are largely non-skilled, lack health insurance, and provide little opportunity for personal growth or development. Indeed, labor and workforce issues are at the center of the system of poverty, poor health, and lack of access to care. In the case of the undocumented, employers may be complicit in the exploitation of a low-wage class of workers who have limited social and workplace rights. As a result, over 25% of recent Mexican immigrants and nearly 20% of long-stay Mexican immigrants live with incomes below the poverty line and have associated lower access to health care and other negative effects on their health status.

Mexican Immigrants in the United States—Access to Care

Among Latinos, Mexicans are one of the most disadvantaged groups in terms of access to care. A series of barriers, of which poverty, lack of insurance, and cultural and linguistic barriers are the most prominent, prevent Mexican immigrants from seeking health services.

Health insurance

Latinos have lower rates of health insurance than other ethnic groups, with Mexican immigrants facing the greatest burden (**Fig. 1**). Parallel to the growth of Mexican migration, the size of the uninsured Mexican population more than doubled over the past 13 years from 3.3 to 6.7 million people. Today, 56% of the Mexican immigrant population lacks any kind of health insurance coverage. This situation is particularly dramatic among recent arrivals in the United States. Those with fewer than 10 years of residence in the country have vulnerability rates (lack of health insurance) of approximately 70%, whereas those who have lived in the United States for over 10 years have vulnerability rates that are 20% to 30% lower.

One of the greatest factors causing the low rates of health insurance among Mexican immigrants is the lack of employer-based insurance. In the United States, most health insurance is provided by employers, yet for the low-paid immigrant workers, this is rarely the case. The major industries that provide significant employment opportunities for the US Mexican labor force include agricultural, manufacturing, construction, and service sectors (**Fig. 2**). They are not only low-paying industries, but also less likely to provide health insurance coverage and other employer-sponsored benefits for their employees. Furthermore, the low incomes make it difficult, if not impossible, for individuals to purchase private health insurance.

Social Determinants of Health

The economic and social conditions in which Mexican immigrants in the United States live determine in great part their access to health services and ultimately their health status. Among these are poverty, documentation status, and cultural and linguistic barriers.

Poverty

The inability to pay for health services is frequently noted as a primary reason for limiting or avoiding all together medical care. It is therefore not surprising that noncitizens of Mexican or Central or South American origin, who are the among the poorest immigrant groups in the United States, are twice as likely to report having no regular source of care as their naturalized counterparts (**Fig. 3**).[16] In addition, basic necessities to keep families healthy, including adequate housing, nutritious food, and needed medical care, including preventive services, are hard to attain with limited incomes.

Documentation status

The many undocumented Mexican immigrants in the United States face even greater barriers to health insurance. For the native-born citizen in financial need, the US health system designates limited funds to providing health coverage to the most vulnerable; however, immigrant families are often not eligible for these programs. It is estimated that undocumented migrants make up 15% of the total uninsured population in the United States, accounting for approximately 6.8 million people. Moreover, increasing anti-immigrant sentiments and policies in the United States are further limiting the resources available to noncitizens, and at the same time making people more fearful of seeking services.

Cultural and linguistic barriers: one size does not fit all

Along with a lack of health coverage, there are several additional barriers to care. These include lack of knowledge of available services and lack of comfort with health care services/facilities.[17] More than 1 in 10 US residents now speak Spanish at home, and approximately half of these persons report they speak English less than 'very well'.[18] While attempts have been made to increase bilingual services, cultural

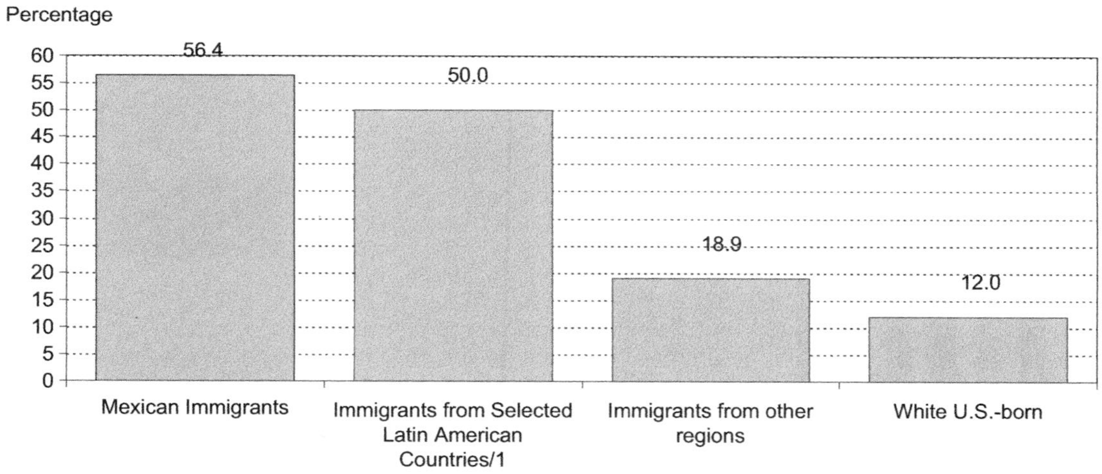

Source: CONAPO estimates, based on *Current Population Survey* (CPS), March 2007 supplement.

Fig. 1. Immigrant population and white U.S.-born population without medical insurance in United States, 2007. *Courtesy of* Health Initiative of the Americas, University of California at Berkeley, School of Public Health, Berkeley, CA; with permission.

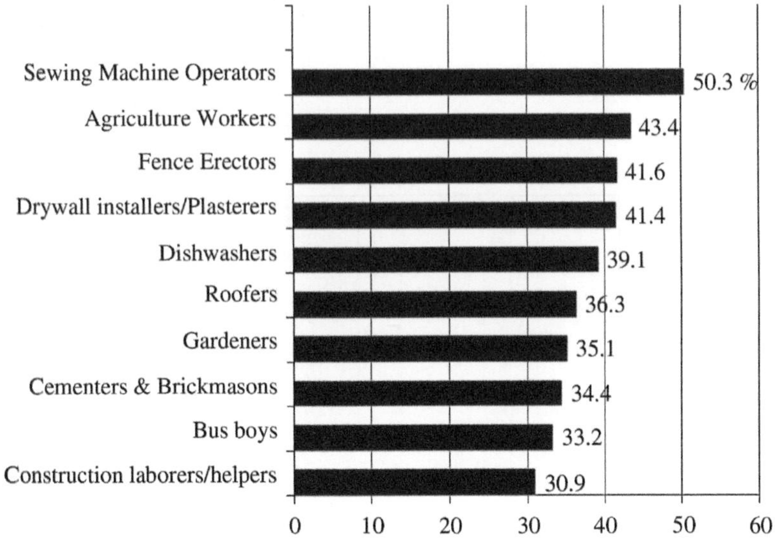

Source: CONAPO Estimates based on U.S. Census Bureau, 2006 Current Population Survey

Fig. 2. Mexican immigrants (males) as percent of all workers per occupation. U.S labor force, 2006. *Courtesy of* Health Initiative of the Americas, University of California at Berkeley, School of Public Health, Berkeley, CA; with permission.

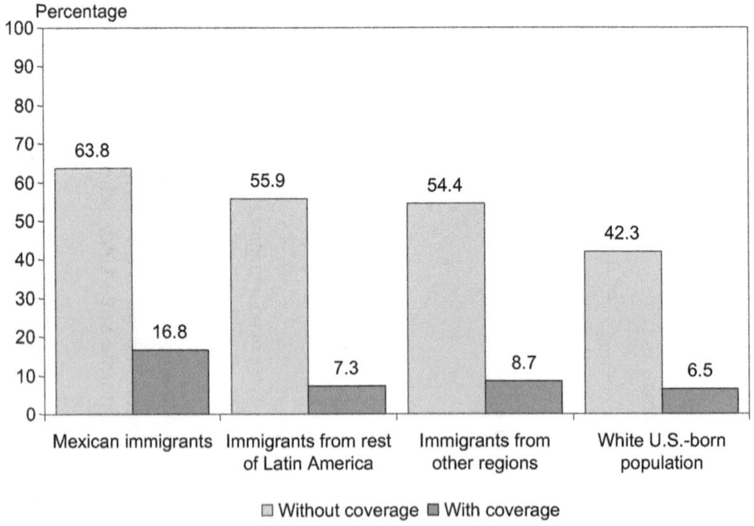

Source: CONAPO estimates, based on *National Health Interview Survey* (NHIS), 2006.

Fig. 3. Immigrant population (from mexico and other regions) and white U.S.-born population with no place for regular medical care in United States by medical security coverage, 2006. *Courtesy of* Health Initiative of the Americas, University of California at Berkeley, School of Public Health, Berkeley, CA; with permission.

sensitivity continues to be a barrier. The under-representation of Latino health care professionals and culturally sensitive professionals in general is a great barrier to care. Providers are often times unaware of the cultural differences between themselves and their patients, creating an environment conducive to mistrust and even fear.

Mexican Immigrants in the United States—Health Status

While much of the data around Mexican immigrants do not address gender differences, it is important to understand each group individually. Women, for example, have different experiences, as well as different health needs and vulnerabilities. It is essential to understand biological, gender, environmental, social, cultural, and economic differences between men and women, which influence their state of health, their search for health care, and their utilization patterns. For example, women's reproductive health needs; their higher prevalence rates of certain chronic diseases; and their greater life expectancy, coupled with changing gender roles brought on by migration, call for more in-depth knowledge addressing their particular needs in terms of health and well-being.

Mexican Immigrant Women in the United States

Mexican-born women constitute the largest female immigrant group in the United States (5 times larger than the second largest, Filipina immigrants) (**Fig. 4**). They account for approximately 46% of the nearly 12 million Mexican migrants in the United States. Most characterized by low educational attainment, limited English proficiency, low naturalization rates, low participation in the formal work force, and living in low-income households. All of these characteristics have negative implications for their health.

Access to health insurance and health services

Over half (52.3%) of all adult Mexican immigrant women in the United States are not covered by some health insurance system, a figure lower than for other immigrant women (**Fig. 5**). Consequently, nearly one-third of them do not have a usual source

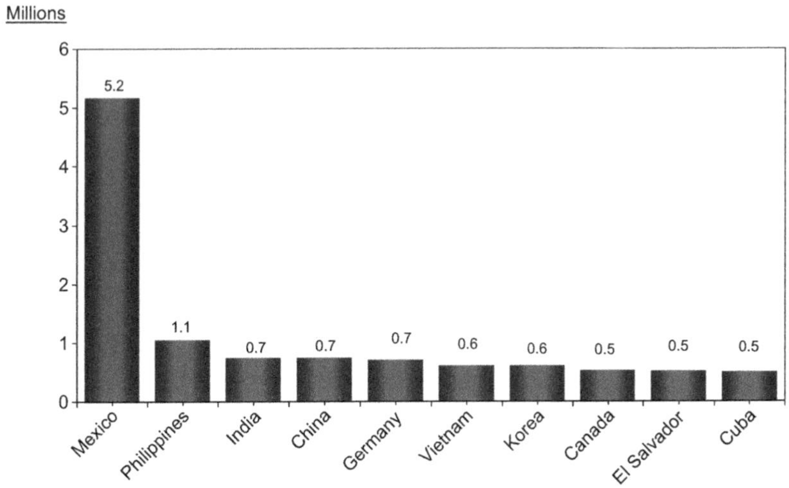

Source: CONAPO estimates based on *American Community Survey (ACS)*,2008.

Fig. 4. Main countries of origin of female immigrant population in United States. *Courtesy of* Health Initiative of the Americas, University of California at Berkeley, School of Public Health, Berkeley, CA; with permission.

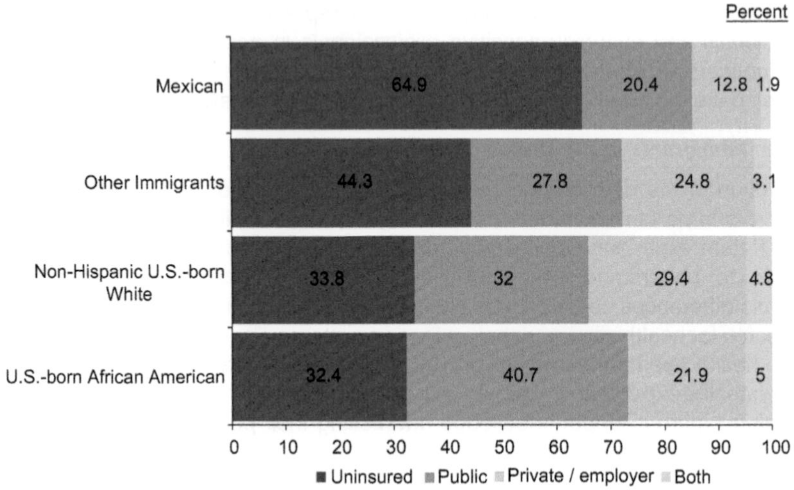

Notes: 1/ Income below 150% of U.S. Federal Poverty Line.

Source: CONAPO estimates based on Current Population Survey (CPS), March 2009.

Fig. 5. Women ages 18 to 64 living in the U.S, with low incomes1, by type of medical insurance and race/ethnicity, 2009. *Courtesy of* Health Initiative of the Americas, University of California at Berkeley, School of Public Health, Berkeley, CA; with permission.

of care and have much lower utilization of prevention services compared with other women in the United States. Those with a regular source of health care are less likely to be attended by private physicians, and instead use public centers or clinics.

Health status

In general, Mexican immigrant women have better health than other immigrant and US-born women, but this advantage disappears with increased time living in the United States. Further, a detailed analysis reveals considerable differences in the prevalence of certain preventable, so-called lifestyle diseases. For instance, diabetes, including gestational diabetes, is more common among Mexican immigrant women. Similarly, Mexican-born women are more likely to be overweight or obese than other immigrant or US-born white women, and they are also more likely to suffer from disorders related to being overweight.

Of great concern for the health of women themselves and for future generations is a lack of prenatal care among this population. Mexican-born mothers are less likely to receive prenatal care in the first trimester of pregnancy than other immigrants and US-born whites. Even more alarming, 7% of Mexican immigrant women who gave birth began receiving health care during the last months of pregnancy, and 3% did not visit a doctor during their entire pregnancy.

The United States provides a number of programs for pregnant women regardless of documentation status, services that are not being used. Whether it is for a lack of information, language barriers, or cultural differences, more needs to be understood about this situation. The health of the children of immigrants demands special attention, as they are the face of the nation's future and thus manifest the future health of the nation.

The Children of Mexican Immigrants

As a result of increased immigration from all countries, the children of immigrants constitute a key segment of the young population in the United States, representing approximately 24% of the total number of children in the country. In other words, nearly 1 out of every 4 children under 18 in the United States has at least one immigrant parent. The number of children with parents from Mexico is particularly high, equal to 6.3 million or 39% of the total number of all children with immigrant parents and close to the total number of African-American children in the United States (**Fig. 6**).

Many of the 6.3 million children of Mexican immigrants in the United States are under 6 years old (38%), while 62% are ages 6 to 17. Most born in the United States (86%), and only 14% were born in Mexico. As one would expect, the proportion of those born in the United States is higher among children under the age of 6 (95%). One would also expect that because these children were born in the United States, they have US citizens' rights and thus full access to health insurance and health services. Nevertheless, because most of these children are from households where neither parent has US citizenship (59.8%) (**Fig. 7**), they often reflect the disadvantaged situation of their parents. The aforementioned barriers to care (ie, documentation status, cultural and language barriers, poverty) prevent the children of Mexican immigrants from fully accessing their US. citizenship rights.

Access to health insurance and health services

In the United States, nearly 1 out of every 10 children under 18 (6.2 million) is not covered by a health insurance system. Within this group, the children of Mexican immigrants are over-represented. While they account for 9% of all children in the country, they constitute 24% of uninsured children, approximately 1.5 million. Within this group are many US-born children of Mexicans; they are far less likely than any other ethnic or racial group to have health insurance coverage. One of every 5 lacks health insurance, whereas in the case of the children of immigrants of other regions and US-born whites and African Americans, this proportion is less than 1 in 10 (**Fig. 8**). Moreover, the children of Mexican immigrants are less likely to have private

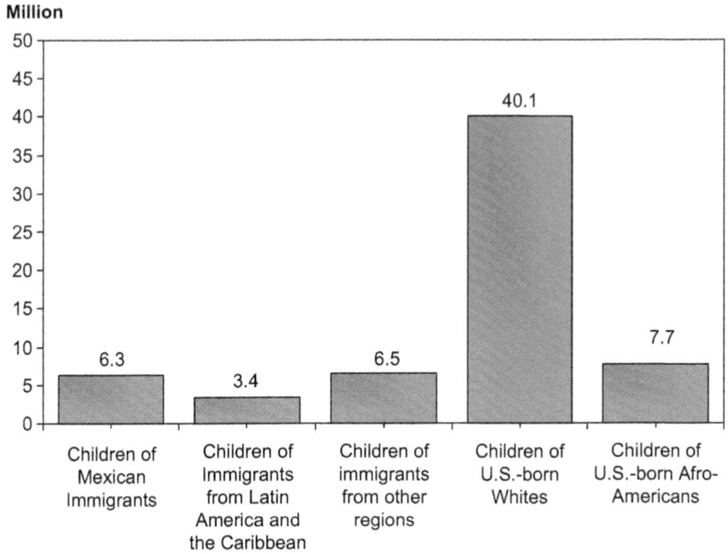

Source: CONAPO estimates based on *Current Population Survey (CPS)*, March 2008.

Fig. 6. Children under 18 in United States by parents' region of origin and ethnicity/race, 2008. *Courtesy of* Health Initiative of the Americas, University of California at Berkeley, School of Public Health, Berkeley, CA; with permission.

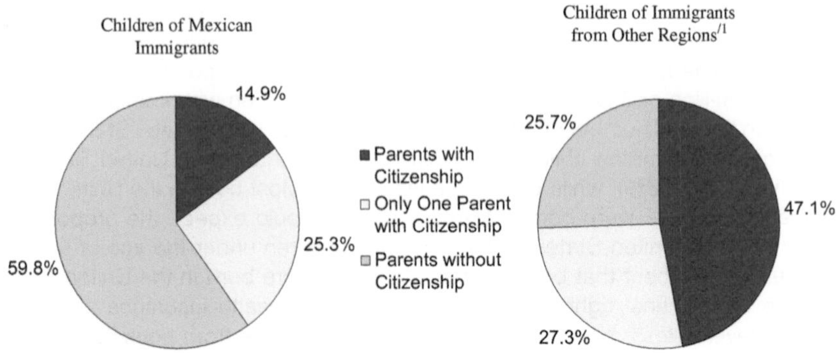

Notes: 1/Excludes immigrants born in Latin America and the Caribbean.
Source: CONAPO estimates based on *Current Population Survey (CPS)*, March 2008.

Fig. 7. Children under 18 of immigrants in United States by citizenship status and parents' region of origin, 2008. *Courtesy of* Health Initiative of the Americas, University of California at Berkeley, School of Public Health, Berkeley, CA; with permission.

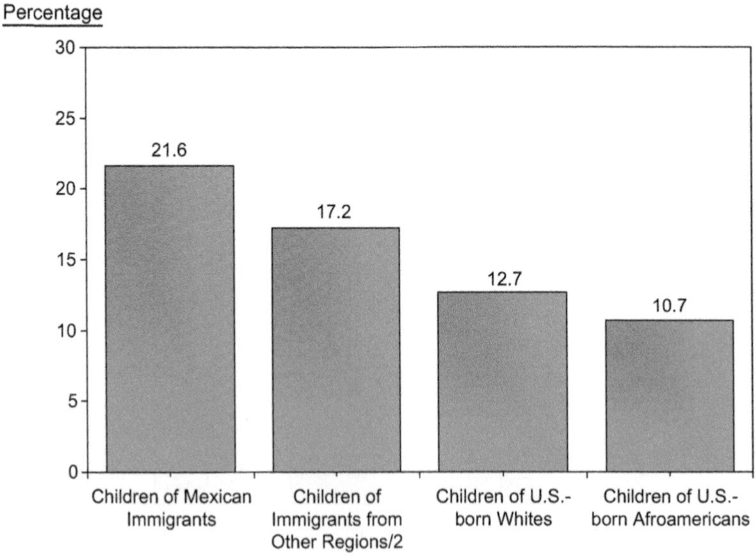

Notes: 1/ Income below 150% of Federal Poverty Line
2/ Excludes Immigrants born in Latin America and the Caribbean.
Source: CONAPO estimates based on Census Bureau, Current Population Survey (CPS), March 2008

Fig. 8. Distribution of U.S-Born children under 18 in United States in limited income families1 without health insurance by parents' region of origin and ethnic group/race, 2008. *Courtesy of* Health Initiative of the Americas, University of California at Berkeley, School of Public Health, Berkeley, CA; with permission.

health insurance and face more obstacles to access to public health programs due to their parents' situation (ie, lack of information, language barriers, and fear of accessing programs due to deportation). Consequently, Mexican immigrant children are less likely to meet the recommended schedule of doctor visits, and less likely to have a regular source of care (**Fig. 9**).

The proportion of Mexican immigrant children ages 2 to 17 who did not visit a doctor over the past year (1 of every 5) is double that of children of immigrants from other regions, as well as that of children of US-born whites and African Americans (approximately 1 in 10). Thus, they are more exposed to the risks posed by not dealing with illnesses at the time they occur. Developmental problems may also be detected later, which, in the long run, may affect children's physical and academic performance and make them more vulnerable to a number of health-related disorders and problems. It is alarming that 1 out of every 20 children of Mexican immigrants (under age 18) has never visited a doctor in the United States.

Health status

Studies indicate that Mexican children do not appear to have worse health than other children per se, but they do have a demographic profile that calls for more attention (see **Fig. 6**). Furthermore, under-diagnosis due to low utilization of health services could be masking the real health status of these children.

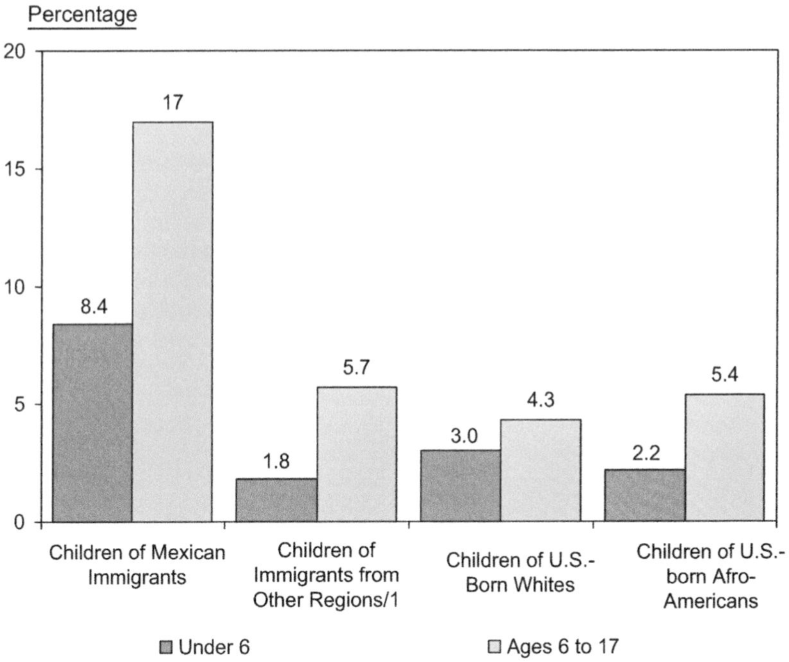

Notes: 1/ Excludes population born in Latin America and the Caribbean.
Source: CONAPO estimates based on *National Health Interview Survey*, 2006-2008.

Fig. 9. Children in the United States without a place for regular medical care by age group, region of origin and parents' ethnic group/race, 2006–2008. *Courtesy of* Health Initiative of the Americas, University of California at Berkeley, School of Public Health, Berkeley, CA; with permission.

Mexican children in the United States are more likely to suffer from anemia, diarrhea. and colitis, suggesting that one of the most common problems of these children is malnutrition. Among children under 3, the prevalence of attacks or convulsions is also higher than among children of other groups. Additionally, the children of Mexicans have a high incidence of low and high birth weight, and are disproportionately affected by 2 of today's biggest health concerns: obesity/overweight and diabetes. Van Hook and colleagues found that beginning with the fourth year of elementary school, over 40% of US-born Latino children suffer from being overweight or obesity, with boys at particularly high risk of being overweight.[19] In addition, Healthy People 2010 reported that Latino children are disproportionately affected by oral disease. Among children aged 6 to 8 years, 43% of Latino children and 36% of non-Latino black children had untreated caries, compared with 26% of non-Latino white children.

The prevalence of so-called lifestyle diseases among women and children reflects in part their disadvantaged position in the United States. These are ailments that could be prevented with proper education and care including regular medical check-ups, proper nutrition, and regular exercise, among others, all of which require luxuries (ie, time, money) that are not easily available for low-income populations. Mexican parents who work in the most demanding jobs or in two jobs have little time and money to engage in some of these preventive measures, and for the undocumented, the fear of repercussion may keep them from seeking available services.

SUMMARY

The situation of Mexican immigrants in the United States reflects inequalities and gaps in the current health system as well as in society overall. Most Mexican immigrants do not have access to health insurance or health services or adequate housing, and they work and live under conditions detrimental to their health and well-being. They are disproportionately affected by lifestyle conditions such as diabetes, overweight/obesity, and poor oral health among others, which point to factors associated with their immigration status, including lower education levels, poverty, and unhealthy living environment. Yet, the disadvantaged health status of immigrants in the United States is not exclusive to Mexican immigrants; it is an issue relevant to those from many other regions of the world.

Migration is a global phenomenon that has existed for centuries and will continue to exist in the future. Even though the topic of migration and health has gained more interest in the last decade, it is still an area where academics and health professionals require more training and education, especially in regards to health promotion, to conduct better research and offer more effective interventions. In addition, enlightened policies are needed to address the unique health needs of this population. As economic and social inequalities among nations and the demand for labor continue, the scope of migration will continue to grow. The health concerns of migrants are no longer minority issues; they are major demographic shifts affecting the countries of origin and receiving countries. Immigrants in the United States deserve recognition for their many contributions and should no longer be seen as the other. In the case of Latinos, both the United States and Latin American countries should recognize and acknowledge their role in the migration process and take the responsibility for the health and human rights of the millions who cross the border each year hoping to find better opportunities on the other side.

ACKNOWLEDGMENTS

The authors would like to thank and acknowledge the National Population Council of Mexico (CONAPO) for valuable contributions to the Migration and Health Issues Reports, which made a large part of this article possible.

REFERENCES

1. López-Acuña D, Mosca D, Pace P, et al. Health of migrants: the way forward. World Health Organization report. Madrid (Spain): World Health Organization; 2010.
2. Barnett ED, Walker PF. Role of immigrants and migrants in emerging infectious diseases. Med Clin North Am 2008;92:1447–58.
3. Field V, Gautret P, Schlagenhauf P, et al. Travel and migration associated infectious diseases morbidity in Europe, 2008. BMC Infect Dis 2010;10:330.
4. Misra A, Ganda OP. Migration and its impact on adiposity and type 2 diabetes. Nutrition 2007;23:696–708.
5. Immigration, health and work: the facts behind the myths. Available at: http://hia.berkeley.edu/index.php?page=migration-and-health-reports. Accessed November 22, 2010.
6. Latinos in the United States, 2008. Available at: http://hia.berkeley.edu/index.php?page=migration-and-health-reports. Accessed November 22, 2010.
7. The children of Mexican immigrants in the US. Available at: http://hia.berkeley.edu/index.php?page=migration-and-health-reports. Accessed November 22, 2010.
8. Mexican immigrant women in the U.S. Available at: http://hia.berkeley.edu/index.php?page=migration-and-health-reports. Accessed November 22, 2010.
9. United Nations international migrant stock, 2008 revision. Available at: http://esa.un.org/migration. Accessed November 5, 2010.
10. Grieco E. Race and Hispanic origin of the foreign-born population in the United States, 2007. American Community Survey Reports, US Census; January 2010. Available at: http://www.census.gov/prod/2010pubs/acs-11.pdf. Accessed December 4, 2010.
11. Hoefer M, Rytina N, Baker BC. Estimates of the unauthorized Immigrant population in the United States: January 2008. Office of Immigration Statistics, Policy Directorate, US Department of Homeland Security; 2009. Available at: http://www.dhs.gov/xlibrary/assets/statistics/publications/ois_ill_pe_2008.pdf. Accessed November 1, 2010.
12. US Census: fact finder. Available at: http://factfinder.census.gov/servlet/ACSSAFFFacts?_submenuId=factsheet_1&_sse=on. Accessed December 14, 2010.
13. Grieco E. Race and hispanic origin of the foreign-born population in the United States, 2007. American Community Survey Reports. 2010. Available at: http://www.census.gov/prod/2010pubs/acs-11.pdf. Accessed December 14, 2010.
14. Pew Hispanic Center (fact sheet) Hispanics of Mexican origin in the United States. Available at: http://pewhispanic.org/files/factsheets/59.pdf. Accessed January 10, 2011.
15. Castañeda X, Wallace SP, Guendelman S. Immigration, health and work: the facts behind the myths. Migration and Health Report, Health Initiative of the Americas. UC Berkeley, Berkeley CA; 2007. Available at: http://hia.berkeley.edu/index.php?page5migration-and-health-reports. Accessed November 4, 2010.
16. Callahan ST, Hickson GB, Cooper WO. Health care access of Hispanic young adults in the United States. J Adolesc Health 2006;39(5):627–33.
17. Castañeda X, Ojeda G. Access to health care for Latinos in the US (online fact sheet). Health Initiative of the Americas. University of California Berkeley, School of Public Health. Berkeley, CA; 2010. Available at: http://hia.berkeley.edu/uploads/accesstohealthcare_factsheet.pdf. Accessed December 14, 2010.
18. DuBard CA, Gizlice Z. Language spoken and differences in health status, access to care, and receipt of preventive services among US Hispanics. Am J Public Health 2008;98(1):2021–8.
19. Van Hook J, Balistreri KS, Baker E. Moving to the land of milk and cookies: obesity among the children of immigrants. Migration Information Source, Migration Policy Institute. Washington, DC; 2009.

REFERENCES

Global Health: Governance and Policy Development

Patrick W. Kelley, MD, DrPH

KEYWORDS

• Global health • Governance • Policy • Globalization

Collective global action is increasingly recognized as central to achieving the highest attainable standard of health and wellbeing for the world's people. Governance constitutes the constellation of mechanisms a society uses to effect collective action toward common goals. Although individuals bear the major responsibility for maintaining healthy lifestyles and for seeking appropriate preventive and therapeutic care, many factors necessary for health can only be established through collective action on a larger scale.

Effective collective action requires coordinated policy and a collaborative approach to implementation. Historically, the purview of sovereign states and intergovernmental organizations like the World Health Organization (WHO), global health policy is now being influenced by an ever-increasing number of nonstate and non-intergovernmental actors with a range of mandates, interests, resources, means, and degrees of accountability.

Illustrative community needs amenable to organized, collective public-health solutions include the need to provide individuals with access to safe, potable water, hygienic housing and worksites, nutritious and uncontaminated food and drugs, and protection from infectious diseases. In recent decades, the challenges for global health governance have grown to encompass the prevention of interpersonal violence, unintentional injuries, threats to mental and reproductive health, and the prevention of global epidemics of chronic diseases. In health systems, current challenges include addressing the consequences of health-workforce migrations from communities in dire need to meet the growing demand for health workers in wealthier countries. Increases in global trade have extended the public-health mandate to concern about the safety and effectiveness of imported food, pharmaceuticals, and other products.

The author has nothing to disclose except that his organization has grants and contracts with many of the donor organizations cited in this article.

Disclaimer: Unless otherwise referenced, the opinions herein are those of the author alone and should not be construed as representing the position of the Institute of Medicine or the National Academies.

Boards on Global Health and African Science Academy Development, Institute of Medicine, National Academies, 500 Fifth Street North West, Washington, DC 20001, USA

E-mail address: pkelley@nas.edu

Infect Dis Clin N Am 25 (2011) 435–453
doi:10.1016/j.idc.2011.02.014 id.theclinics.com

Threats to health, actual and perceived, can also constitute challenges to peace, economic prosperity, family and military stability, and human rights. Responding to health threats can bring into tension competing global interests that require resolution in the global governance arena (eg, reconciling the right to have access to lifesaving antiretroviral drugs with intellectual property regimes). Indeed, many public goods can now be achieved only with global collective action.

GLOBALIZATION: A DRIVER FOR GLOBAL HEALTH GOVERNANCE

In the mid-nineteenth century there was recognition that collective supranational action was needed to control epidemic diseases, such as plague and cholera. From 1851 to 1903, at least 11 international sanitary conferences were convened to address the threats of cholera, yellow fever, and plague.[1] The motivation for these conferences was not merely the protection of individual health but also the implementation of disease control so that the benefits of industrialization, global trade, and cross-border traffic would not be unduly hampered.

The geo-temporal challenge of global health governance in the nineteenth century was modest. In 1850, when the world population was about 1.2 billion, an individual needed about 1 year to circumnavigate the globe. By 2000, when the world population had increased to more than 6 billion, a determined traveler could cover the same distance in less than 48 hours.[2] Pathogens can now be carried far and wide with great rapidity, as was seen with severe acute respiratory syndrome (SARS) in 2003 and with the H1N1 pandemic in 2009.[3,4]

In the twenty-first century, the health impacts of globalization go far beyond the international spread of naturally occurring emerging infections.[5] Medically inappropriate or inadequate uses of antimicrobial drugs have hastened the spread of resistant organisms (eg, extremely drug-resistant tuberculosis), which can migrate and threaten even well-developed countries. Sadly, biologic and chemical terrorism are ongoing threats, despite the provisions of the Biologic and Chemical Weapons Conventions.[6] Two perhaps less-obvious phenomena are the globalization of pharmaceuticals and food supplies.

Pharmaceuticals originating in many developing countries have been associated with a range of quality problems, yet they are increasingly imported to the United States. According to calculations based on the United Nations (UN) Commodity Trade Statistics Database, the dollar value of pharmaceuticals imports to the United States from all parts of the world increased more than 22-fold between 1985 and 2005. During that same period, when the values of imports from Switzerland and the United Kingdom increased 11-fold and 12-fold, respectively, the comparable increases for imports from China and India were 23-fold and 65-fold, respectively.[7] Some pharmaceutical-manufacturing problems in the developing world may even reflect intentional adulteration. In 2007 and 2008 exported heparin of Chinese origin that included oversulfated chondroitin sulfate was tied to 149 US deaths in which one or more allergic/hypotensive symptoms were reported.[8] The pharmaceutical-import business is so large that the US Food and Drug Administration (FDA) inspection of products at US points of entry is logistically impractical.

As depicted in **Fig. 1**, the globalization of agricultural trade over the last several decades has also been remarkable. Excluding imports from Canada and 27 nations of the European Union, the dollar value of agricultural imports to the United States from the next 13 national sources totaled about $32,808,623,000 in 2009. Of this, approximately 51% was attributable to trade with Mexico, China, Brazil, Thailand, and India.[9] A 2008 US Government Accountability Office report estimated that at

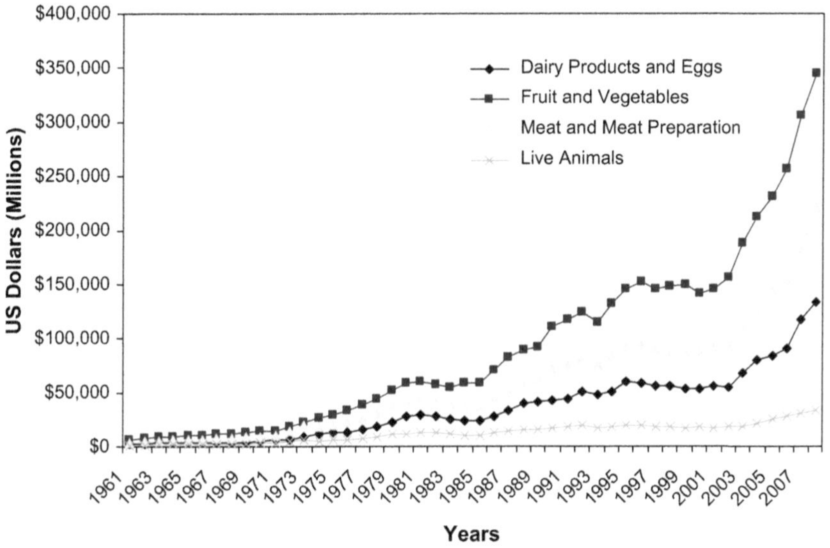

Fig. 1. Trends in international agricultural trade (total world imports + total world exports) by commodity type, 1961 to 2008. (*Data from* FAOSTAT, Statistics Division, Food and Agriculture Organization of the UN. Available at: http://faostat.fao.org/site/535/default.aspx#ancor, http://faostat.fao.org/site/604/default.aspx#ancor. Accessed March 23, 2011.)

recent inspection rates it would cost the FDA $3.16 billion and take more than 13 years to inspect the 189,000 foreign facilities involved with registered food production for export to the United States.[10]

Governance structures for building consensus and for collectively managing public health actions are necessary because the world's inhabitants cannot create societies and economies that are largely self-contained and insulated from outside threats. The world's inhabitants increasingly share the same air, water, exposure to infectious diseases, foods, pharmaceuticals, and health workforce. Through climate change, the impact of human activities in a few countries can affect harvests, the epidemiology of infectious diseases, and the potential for global natural disasters.[11] Even among countries with strong public health programs, harmonization of standards and processes is important for effective and efficient collective action. Today's global health governance structures include a complex web of UN agencies, public/private partnerships, donor and recipient governments, foundations, corporations, and civil society organizations. A recent report from the Kaiser Family Foundation identified 50 multilateral international health treaties, commitments, partnerships, and other agreements, 26 of which are legally binding under international law. The United States is a party to 36 of these of agreements, 16 of which are legally binding. These agreements cover many topical areas, including specific diseases, environmental issues, trade and intellectual property, specific populations (eg, refugees or children), health security/preparedness, water, and food/nutrition.[12]

THE CURRENT ARCHITECTURE OF GLOBAL HEALTH GOVERNANCE

The World Health Organization and Other United Nations Agencies

In the aftermath of the nineteenth-century international sanitary conferences that focused on threats to ports and trade, the early twentieth century saw international global health governance reflected in new institutions, such as the International Sanitary Bureau (ISB) based in Washington, DC, and the Office Internationale d'Hygiéne Publique in Paris. The ISB subsequently became the Pan American Health Organization, which since 1948 has been one of 6 regional offices of the WHO. When the UN system was conceived in 1945, Brazil and China proposed the WHO. The WHO constitution contains several key principles, including:

> *Health is a state of complete physical, mental and social well-being and not merely the absence of disease or infirmity.*
>
> *The enjoyment of the highest attainable standard of health is one of the fundamental rights of every human being without distinction of race, religion, political belief, economic or social condition.*
>
> *The health of all peoples is fundamental to the attainment of peace and security and is dependent upon the fullest co-operation of individuals and States.*[13]

The broad mandate of the WHO has 6 core functions: the provision of collective health leadership, the shaping of research as well as the generation and dissemination of knowledge, the setting of norms and standards and the promotion and monitoring of their implementation, the production of ethical and evidence-based policy options, the provision of technical support and capacity-building, and the monitoring of health situations and trends.[14] The organization has a 6-point agenda: promote development; foster health security; strengthen health systems; harness research, information, and evidence; enhance partnerships; and improve performance.[15] This agenda is shaped at annual meetings in Geneva by the 193 member countries that compose the World Health Assembly. An 8000-person secretariat based in Geneva and at the 6 regional and 147 country offices performs WHO programs. The breadth of the programs undertaken is vast, although not always deep. Some of the topics addressed include HIV/AIDS; malaria; tuberculosis; chronic noncommunicable diseases; mental disorders; violence; traffic safety; visual impairment; maternal and child health; aging; disasters; health equity; environmental health; nutrition and food safety; drug access; research; health systems strengthening; and tobacco, alcohol, and drug abuse, and other unsafe behaviors.

When the WHO was envisioned, the concept of its operations was quite vertical and focused primarily on relationships with member states. Few other actors were engaged in global health. Since its founding, the WHO has celebrated major accomplishments but has also suffered from an erosion of its influence. Beyond the eradication of smallpox (an event that has likely saved more than 20 million lives since 1977), WHO technical leadership has also played a role in the near eradication of polio; the containment of the deadly 2003 SARS epidemic; the landmark 2003 WHO Framework Convention on Tobacco Control (the first treaty negotiated under the auspices of WHO); and the 2005 revision of the International Health Regulations (IHR). Compared with the previous IHR that was focused on classical diseases of international importance, plague, yellow fever, and cholera, the 2005 revision is more powerful and practical in that it encompasses all acute public health risks of transnational significance. The new IHR defines broad reporting requirements and establishes the authority of the WHO to initiate disease-control actions, if necessary, through use of information sources other than country governments. The new IHR also requires countries to strengthen their existing surveillance capacities.

Many have hoped that the WHO would take a stronger role in the setting and enforcement of norms, given its extraordinary constitutional authorities and its quasi-legislative power to adopt binding regulations. The WHO has, however, leaned more toward providing technical advice than toward exerting bold, proactive leadership through binding norms and regulations.[16]

Given its mandate, the WHO is handicapped by a modest budget and by its dependent fiscal relationships. The proposed budget for 2010 to 2011 was $4.94 billion before currency adjustments. Because only about 18.8% of the WHO budget comes from the dues assessments of member countries, its flexibility in focusing its program based on the scientific priorities it determines is constrained. Wealthier countries pay larger assessments and thus have more influence over the direction of WHO programming than poorer countries, which have the greater need for help. Moreover, the remaining 81.2% of the budget is projected as "voluntary contributions," which are largely earmarked by donors for specific purposes.[17] This arrangement contributes to fragmented programming and perhaps to certain donor-influenced compromises. In this century, the WHO also faces growing challenges. Although its members are sovereign governments, many other powerful actors (including nongovernmental entities, such as other UN agencies, foundations, corporations, and civil society organizations) have entered the global-health arena. Placating these competing interests is not a recipe for bold action.

The United Nation General Assembly and Health

The WHO is the lead UN agency for health. Owing to the increasing recognition that health is fundamental to the broader UN goals of fostering the international rule of law, global security, economic development, social progress, human rights, and world peace, health issues have now taken a more prominent place than they had in the United Nation's first 50 years. In 2001, world leaders came together at the UN headquarters to adopt the 8 Millennium Development Goals (MDGs), 3 of which are focused on health.

The leaders of 192 UN member states agreed to partner to achieve these goals by 2015. The 3 health-related goals have directly provided high-level, consensus global health policy direction (**Box 1**). Another goal is related to hunger reduction. Regrettably, the MDGs lack a target for chronic diseases, such as cardiovascular diseases and cancers, which now account for more than 50% of the global burden of disease.

Since 2000, progress toward the MDG targets has been mixed. For example, between 2003 and 2008, the number of individuals infected with HIV placed on antiretroviral drugs rose from 400,000 to 4 million (ie, 42% of the 8.8 million people in

Box 1
Selected health-related United Nations millennium development goals

Goal 4: Reduce child mortality rate

Target 4A: Reduce the under-5 mortality rate by two-thirds, between 1990 and 2015

Goal 5: Improve maternal health

Target 5A: Reduce the maternal mortality ratio by three-quarters, between 1990 and 2015

Target 5B: Achieve universal access to reproductive health by 2015

Goal 6: Combat HIV/AIDS, malaria, and other diseases

Target 6A: Have halted and begun to reverse the spread of HIV/AIDS by 2015

Target 6B: Achieve universal access to treatment for HIV/AIDS for all those who need it by 2010

Target 6C: Have halted and begun to reverse the incidence of malaria and other major diseases by 2015 need). In developing countries, 37% of births in 2008 still took place without a trained birth attendant present, and maternal mortality remains shockingly high.[18]

As a result of the HIV/AIDS pandemic and its immense scale and impact on human life, dignity, rights, social cohesion, and economic development, a UN General Assembly special session issued a formal Declaration of Commitment on HIV/AIDS in June 2001.[19] That declaration endorsed the establishment of the "Global AIDS and Health Fund," which would pool contributions from countries and from the private sector to fund HIV prevention and treatment efforts. It also set out a policy approach to providing leadership; improving prevention, care, and treatment; preserving human rights; reducing the vulnerability of women and children at risk for or affected by HIV/AIDS; and mobilizing financial resources. A UN special session on noncommunicable diseases and their prevention will convene in September 2011.

As illustrated in **Box 2**, the UN has spawned a wide array of specialized agencies and other entities with direct or indirect interests in health. To some degree, these compete with the WHO for legitimacy and resources, and some have a significant role in global health governance.

In recognition of the multidimensional challenge of HIV/AIDS, the Joint UN Program on HIV/AIDS (UNAIDS) was launched in 1996. Its sponsors are the WHO and 9 other UN entities: the Office of the UN High Commissioner for Refugees (UNHCR); the UN Children's Fund (UNICEF); the World Food Program (WFP); the UN Development Program (UNDP); the UN Population Fund (UNFPA); the UN Office on Drugs and Crime (UNODC); the International Labor Organization (ILO); the UN Educational, Scientific, and Cultural Organization (UNESCO); and the World Bank.

UNAIDS provides coordinated leadership and broad policy guidance on a wide range of areas pertinent to HIV/AIDS. It addresses HIV/AIDS prevention, care, and

Box 2
Major United Nations agencies and organizations with a significant health role

- Food and Agriculture Organization of the United Nations
- International Labor Organization
- Joint United Nations Program on HIV/AIDS
- Organization for the Prohibition of Chemical Weapons
- Office of the UN High Commissioner for Refugees
- United Nations Children's Fund
- United Nations Development Program
- United Nations Development Fund for Women
- United Nations Drug Control Program
- United Nations Educational, Scientific, and Cultural Organization
- United Nations Population Fund
- United Nations World Food Program
- World Bank Group
- World Health Organization
- World Intellectual Property Organization
- World Tourism Organization
- World Trade Organization

treatment, especially among migrants, women and girls, peacekeepers, travelers, and orphans; it unites the relevant UN agencies, civil society organizations, governments, and the private sector; it advocates for rights, resources, and accountability; it empowers actors with strategic information; and it supports country leadership.

Created by the General Assembly in 1946 for post-war relief, UNICEF is now focused on providing on-the-ground, long-term humanitarian and developmental assistance to children and mothers in developing countries. Funded by governments and the private sector, the 2009 UNICEF expenditures totaled $3.3 billion.[20]

Based in Rome, the Food and Agriculture Organization of the United Nations (FAO) operates through regional offices and through more than 70 country offices around the world. With a biennial budget in 2008 to 2009 of $929.8 million, the FAO leads UN efforts to enhance food security and to eliminate hunger, the number-one MDG. The FAO provides a neutral forum in which all countries can negotiate agreements and debate policy. Its experts disseminate technical information and assist countries with disease outbreaks and in developing sound agriculture policies. Where issues of human health and animal health intersect (eg, avian influenza or food safety emergencies), the FAO plays a role.

Although not actually a UN agency, the World Organization for Animal Health (previously known as the Office International des Epizooties and still known as the OIE) is also an intergovernmental organization; it seeks to perform global disease control for the animal population. Based in Paris and having regional and subregional offices worldwide, the OIE is an important partner of the WHO, the FAO, and the World Trade Organization (WTO). Like the WHO, it operates under the collective control and authority of an assembly of member countries. OIE relevance to global health governance stems from the often-underappreciated connection between human health and animal health. This connection, embodied in the one-health concept, is most evident in the context of emerging zoonotic diseases and food safety.[21] In 2009, an Institute of Medicine (IOM) committee concluded that the OIE rules lacked critical provisions found in the 2005 WHO IHR, provisions that would be valuable for an organization involved in protecting animals capable of transmitting infections to humans. The committee recommended that the OIE create legally binding obligations for members to develop and maintain core surveillance-and-response capabilities, that the OIE be authorized to publically disseminate the animal-disease information received from nongovernmental sources when the member state does not do so in a timely and accurate way, and that the OIE director general be empowered to declare animal-health emergencies and related recommendations as appropriate.[22]

The WTO, a member of the UN family since 1995, is primarily concerned with the rules of trade between nations. With globalization, however, trade and health are increasingly connected. The WTO has several agreements related to health and health policies, including the Agreements on Technical Barriers to Trade; the Sanitary and Phytosanitary Measures; the Trade-Related Intellectual Property Rights (TRIPS); and the Trade in Services. Although trade can be restrained for scientifically valid reasons related to health, relevant interpretations can be controversial. Some health issues relevant to WTO agreements include food safety and protection from zoonotic diseases; TRIPS patent protection for pharmaceuticals (to balance incentives for drug development vs ensuring affordable access to drugs); tobacco control; biotechnology; and the transnational migrations of health workers, patients, and investment in health services.[23]

The World Bank Group, founded in 1944, is a critical source of financial and technical help for developing countries. Headquartered in Washington, DC, it employs more than 10,000 people worldwide. The bank provides low-interest loans, interest-free credits, and grants to developing countries for health and other purposes. The World Bank consists primarily of 2 unique development institutions owned by 187 member countries: the International Bank for Reconstruction and Development (IBRD) and the International Development Association (IDA). The IBRD serves middle-income and creditworthy poorer countries; whereas, the IDA mission is to serve the world's poorest countries. IBRD lending is primarily financed through AAA-rated bonds sold on the world's financial markets; the IDA funds come from 40 donor countries and are replenished periodically. Additional funds come from repayments of loan principal on long-term, no-interest loans. The IDA accounts for more than 40% of World Bank lending, and its loans are largely supervised and evaluated by the World Bank country offices. IDA loans have been used to improve sanitation and water supplies, support immunization programs, and combat the HIV/AIDS pandemic.

In fiscal 2009, the World Bank Health, Nutrition, and Population program lent $2.9 billion, a 3-fold increase from 2008. Since 1997, the bank group provided $17 billion in country-level project financing and $873 million in private health and pharmaceutical investments. In fiscal 2009, the bank disbursed $290 million for existing HIV projects and committed nearly $326 million to new HIV/AIDS efforts. It also committed funds in fiscal 2009 for pandemic preparedness.[24]

Bilateral Donor Governments

Achieving the MDGs will require an estimated $20 billion to $70 billion annually.[25] Higher-income countries have made substantial policy commitments to support the lower-income countries that have insufficient resources to provide a basic package of essential health benefits (estimated at $34 per capita per year). Funding for action by wealthier countries has often been coordinated through governance mechanisms, including the annual Group of Eight (G8) summits. G8 progress toward these commitments is summarized in **Table 1**.

In 2002, the UN Millennium Project estimated that to meet the 2015 MDGs, the total overseas development assistance (ODA) from high-income countries would need to

Table 1
Group of Eight progress against key commitments

Commitment	Progress by 2010
Provide at least $60 billion to fight infectious diseases and improve health systems by 2012	The G8 is on track to meet this commitment with 2008 overseas development assistance disbursements exceeding $12 billion.
Provide 100 million insecticide-treated nets for malaria prevention by 2010	The G8 is on track to provide more than 100 million insecticide-treated nets by 2010.
Mobilize support for the Global Fund to Fight AIDS, Tuberculosis, and Malaria (GFATM)	For the 2001 to 2009 period, the G8 contributions, including from the European Commission, to GFATM totaled $12.2 billion, representing 78% of all contributions to the fund.
Support the Global Polio Eradication Initiative	For the period 2005 to 2009, G8 funding to the initiative was $1.68 billion. G8 commitments for the period 2010 to 2012 total $287.4 million.

Data from Muskoka Accountability Report: assessing action and results against development-related commitments (executive summary). 2010. Available at: http://canadainternational.gc.ca/g8/assets/pdfs/muskoka_accountability_report.pdf. Accessed March 22, 2011.

rise to 0.54% of gross national income (GNI). In absolute terms, the US government has contributed great amounts to ODA; however, as depicted in **Fig. 2**, the relative amount contributed in 2009 was only 0.20% of US GNI, a figure less generous than the percentage contributed by most European countries, Australia, and Canada.

The US government's global health program, compared with that of many other donor governments, cuts across many departments. It draws upon both the foreign-assistance structure but also the government's extensive public health capabilities. In addition to well-known actors, such as the US Agency for International Development and the US Centers for Disease Control and Prevention, executive branch agencies with a significant involvement in global health include the departments of state, defense, agriculture, homeland security, labor, and commerce, as well as the National Institutes of Health, the Food and Drug Administration, the Environmental Protection Agency, the Peace Corps, and the Health Resources and Services Administration. These agencies carry out programs in more than 100 countries and are overseen by more than 15 congressional committees.[26]

The US financial commitment to global health has dramatically increased over the last decade, especially with the implementation of the President's Emergency Plan for AIDS Relief (PEPFAR) and the President's Malaria Initiative (**Fig. 3**). Originally authorized in 2003 at about $15 billion, PEPFAR focused on 15 countries, mostly in Africa. Over its first 5 years, PEPFAR sought to support antiretroviral treatment for 2 million people infected with HIV; prevent 7 million HIV infections; and provide care, including care for orphans and vulnerable children, for 10 million individuals. The program has been viewed as a major success for US global health policy.[27] With wide bipartisan support, PEPFAR was reauthorized in 2008 for another 5 years at $39 billion, with substantial increases in the prevention, treatment, and care targets. The legislation also authorized $4 billion for tuberculosis programming and $5 billion for malaria efforts.[28]

Although PEPFAR represents a landmark US achievement in global health, it also illustrates how policy can be skewed by nonscientific factors. **Fig. 4** shows that among

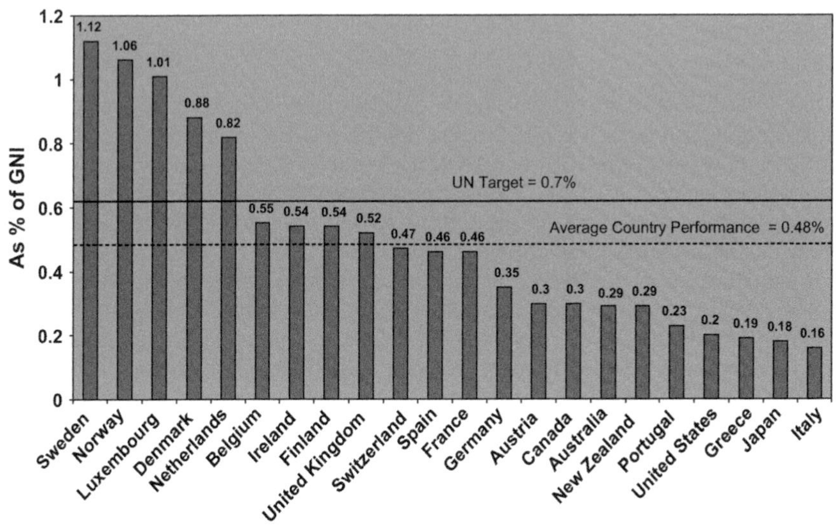

Fig. 2. Net Overseas Development Assistance (ODA) for 2009 as a percent of gross national income. (*Data from* OECD. Chart 1: Net Official Development Assistance in 2009. Available at: http://www.oecd.org/dataoecd/17/9/44981892.pdf. Accessed September 24, 2010.

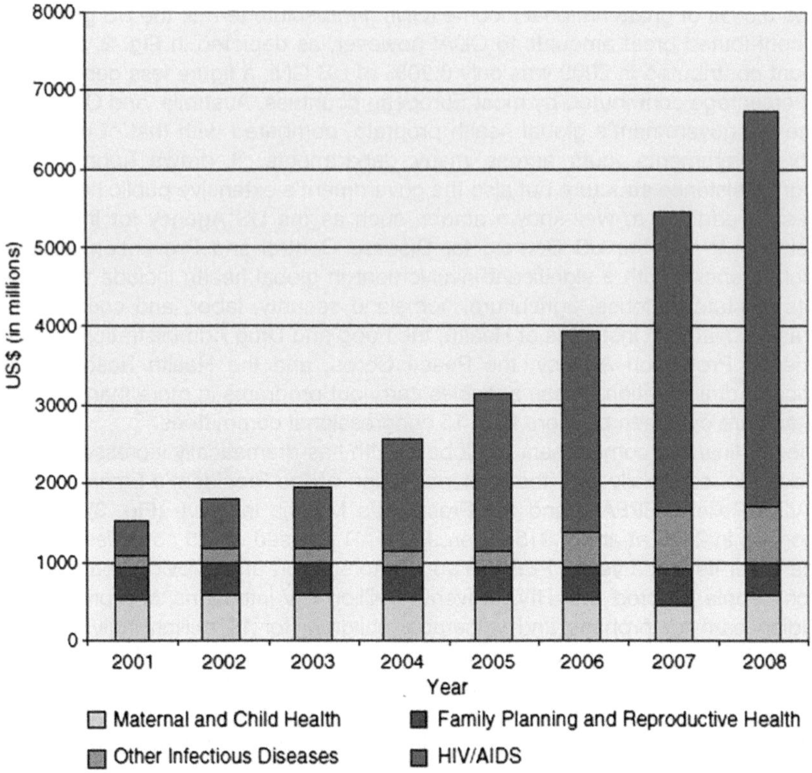

Fig. 3. US State Department (Global HIV/AIDS Initiative) and US Agency for International Development spending on global health (2001–2008). (*From* The Institute of Medicine Committee on the US Commitment to Global Health. The U.S. commitment to global health: recommendations for the public and private sectors. National Academies Press; 2009. p. 137; with permission.)

the top 7 causes of death for individuals younger than 70 years in low-income and middle-income countries, HIV/AIDS accounts for only 8% of those deaths. In fiscal year 2008, however, HIV/AIDS represented more than 52% of the $9.6 billion in US ODA health funding. The 2009 IOM committee on the *US Commitment to Global Health* called for a rebalancing of this portfolio to better support initiatives against non-communicable diseases, malnutrition, and injuries.[29]

The signature global health program of the Obama administration, the Global Health Initiative (GHI), aims to provide $63 billion in health assistance between 2009 and 2014. Although HIV/AIDS still dominates the GHI, increased investments are being made for neglected tropical diseases, malaria, maternal and child health, and family planning (**Box 3**). The aims of the GHI are to implement a woman-centered and girl-centered approach; increase impact and efficiency through strategic coordination and integration; strengthen and leverage key partnerships, multilateral organizations, and private contributions; encourage country ownership and investing in country-led plans; improve metrics, monitoring, and evaluation; and promote research and innovation.[30]

The US government's policy commitment to global health has been greatly lauded as a reflection of our vital health and economic self-interests, our humanitarian values,

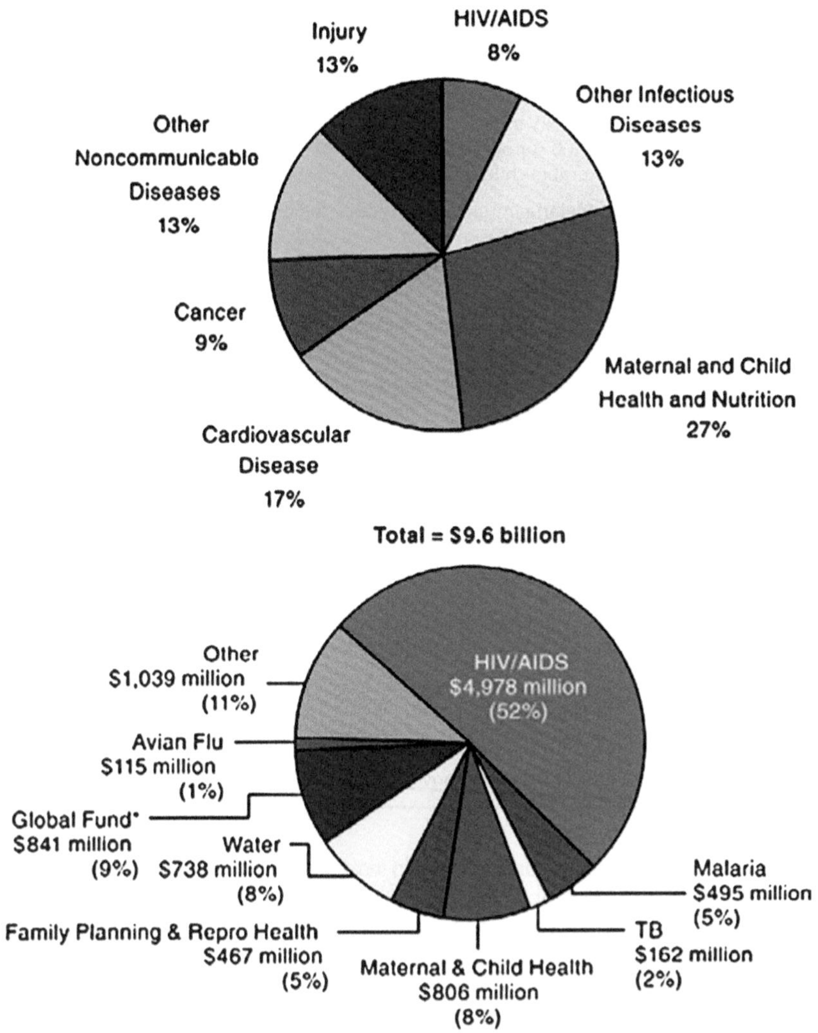

Fig. 4. Leading causes of death in individuals aged younger than 70 years in low-income and middle-income countries versus the distribution of US government funding for global health by major subsector and for the Global Fund, fiscal year 2008. (*From* The Institute of Medicine Committee on the U.S. Commitment to Global Health. The U.S. commitment to global health: recommendations for the public and private sectors. Washington, DC: National Academies Press; 2009. p. 139; with permission.)

and "smart power."[31–33] In many ways, it is an important form of diplomacy; however, some aspects of it may also hinder diplomatic prerogatives. Some forms of ODA can be used as leverage in diplomatic negotiations, but once a patient infected with HIV is taken into a PEPFAR-funded treatment program, it would be unethical for the US government to threaten the loss of those lifesaving drugs for diplomatic advantage.[34]

Public-Private Partnerships

Beyond UN agencies and national governments, the global health enterprise is now a much more horizontal and networked endeavor than it was even 15 years ago.

Box 3
The goals and targets of the US government global health initiative

- HIV/AIDS: The US President's Emergency Plan for AIDS Relief will: (1) support the prevention of more than 12 million new HIV infections; (2) provide direct support for more than 4 million people on treatment; and (3) support care for more than 12 million people, including 5 million orphans and vulnerable children.
- Malaria: The President's Malaria Initiative will reduce the burden of malaria by 50% for 450 million people, representing 70% of the at-risk population in Africa, and expand malaria efforts into Nigeria and the Democratic Republic of the Congo.
- Tuberculosis (TB): Save approximately 1.3 million lives by reducing TB prevalence by 50%, which will involve treating 2.6 million new TB cases and 57,200 multidrug-resistant cases of TB.

Maternal health: Save approximately 360,000 women's lives by reducing maternal mortality by 30% across assisted countries.

- Child health: Save approximately 3 million children's lives, including 1.5 million newborns, by reducing under-5 mortality rates by 35% across assisted countries.
- Nutrition: Reduce child undernutrition by 30% across assisted food-insecure countries, in conjunction with the President's Feed the Future Initiative.
- Family planning and reproductive health: Prevent 54 million unintended pregnancies by meeting unmet need for modern contraception. Contraceptive prevalence is expected to rise to 35% across assisted countries, reflecting an average annual increase of 2 percentage points. First births by women younger than 18 years should decline to 20%.
- Neglected tropical diseases: Reduce the prevalence of 7 neglected tropical diseases by 50% among 70% of the affected population, and eliminate onchocerciasis in Latin America by 2016, lymphatic filariasis globally by 2017, and leprosy.

Data from Available at: http://www.usaid.gov/ghi/factsheet.html.

Although this makes it harder for the WHO to lead, it also brings a wider array of talent and resources to bear on problems. **Fig. 5** illustrates an example of the partnership paradigm of global health governance today: the Roll Back Malaria (RBM) partnership, a 500-member collaboration. Even though the WHO was one of the founders of RBM and hosts the secretariat, it is not positioned as the dominant core of the effort. The RBM partnership not only works to facilitate policy coordination at the global level but also executes an operating framework with performance targets reflective of the MDG malaria goal; it articulates technical strategies and provides multidirectional accountability through its partners forum. A decision-making partnership board with 27 members (6 ex-officio) represents the 7 broad RBM constituencies and meets periodically. There are 21 voting members of the board representing foundations (1 seat), malaria-endemic countries (8 seats), multilateral institutions (4 seats), NGOs (2 seats), Organization for Economic Cooperation and Development (OECD) donor countries (3 seats), private sector (2 seats), and research and academia (1 seat). The Stop TB Partnership (http://www.stoptb.org/) also has many similarities to RBM.

Founded in 2000, the Global Alliance for Vaccines and Immunizations (GAVI) is another innovative partnership that links developing-world governments and donor governments; philanthropic foundations; the financial community; vaccine manufacturers from developed and developing countries; research and technical institutes; civil society organizations; and intergovernmental entities, such as WHO, UNICEF, and the World Bank. Immunizations funded by GAVI have prevented an estimated 3.4 million deaths in developing countries. GAVI also supports innovative financing

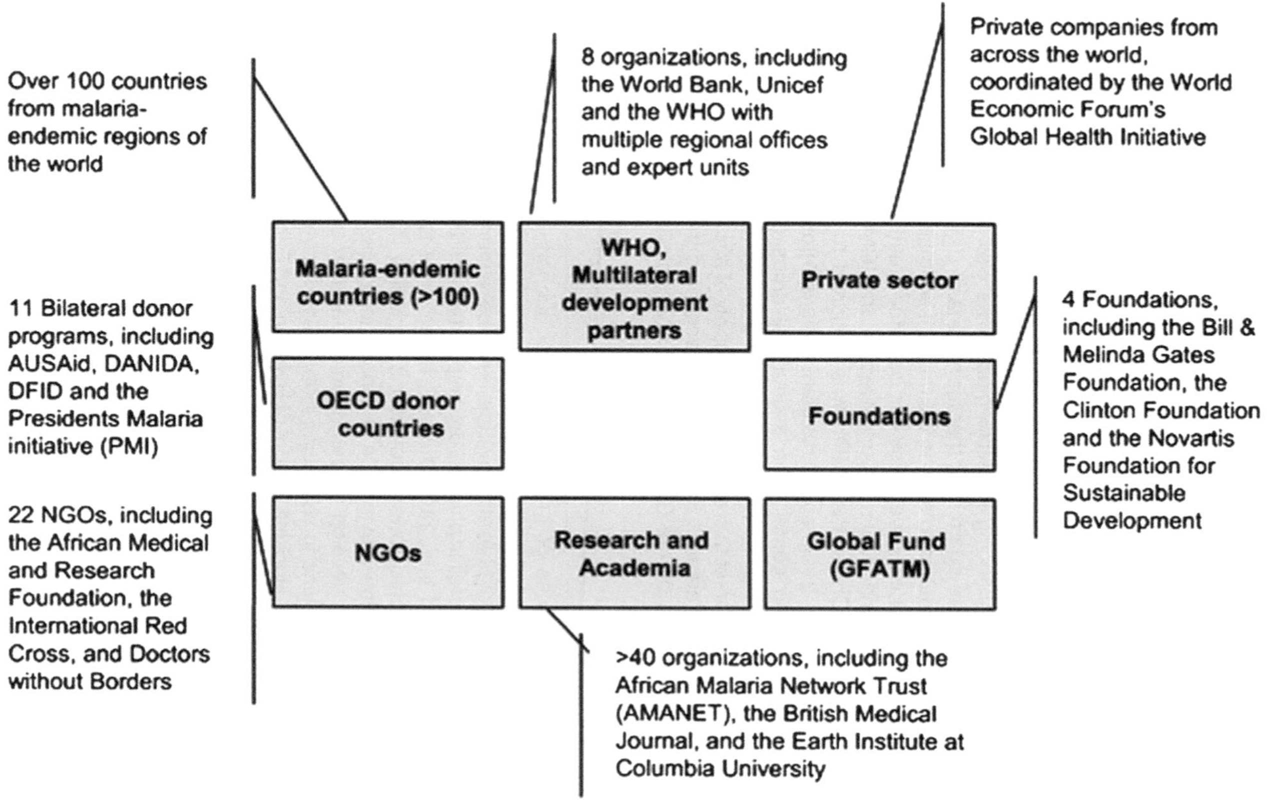

Fig. 5. Roll Back Malaria: Global Health as Partnership. OECD, Organization for Economic Cooperation and Development. AUSAID, Australian Government Overseas AID Program; DANIDA, Danish International Development Agency; DFID, UK Department for International Development. (*From* Szlezák NA, Bloom BR, Jamison DT, et al. The global health system: actors, norms, and expectations in transition. PLoS Med 2010;7(1):e1000183. doi:10.1371/journal.pmed.1000183; with permission.)

mechanisms, such as advanced market commitments to reduce the costs of immunizations needed by developing countries.

The 2001 UN Declaration of Commitment on HIV/AIDS called for the establishment of a global fund of pooled contributions to support HIV/AIDS needs. This Global Fund to Fight AIDS, Tuberculosis, and Malaria (GFATM), unlike the previously mentioned partnerships, has as its sole focus mobilizing and distributing financial resources in a manner driven by technically sound national plans and priorities and principles of transparency and accountability. The GFATM is a partnership between governments, civil society, the private sector, and affected communities. More than 40 countries have pledged funds to the GFATM; other major donors include the Bill and Melinda Gates Foundation, UNITAID, and Chevron. About $21 billion has been pledged, of which more than $16 billion has already been paid.[35] With funding approved for more than 500 programs in nearly 150 countries, the GFATM is the source of one-quarter of all international financing for AIDS globally as well as for two-thirds of that for tuberculosis and three-quarters of that for malaria.[36]

An innovative fiscal contribution to solving the crisis of antimalarial drug resistance and the dwindling number of effective drugs has been the creation of the Affordable Medicines Facility for Malaria (AMFm). Conceived by the IOM Committee on the Economics of Antimalarial Drugs, the AMFm was designed to re-engineer market forces to favor the effective treatment of resistant malaria through the appropriate use of artemisinin-containing combination antimalarial drugs (ACTs). In 2004 the committee recommended the commitment of $300 to $500 million per year to subsidize the entire global ACT market to create a steady supply of affordable and desirably priced ACTs in all malarious areas.[37] Several donors accepted this recommendation. The AMFm was established by the GFATM and initially capitalized with more than $146 million.[35]

Philanthropic Foundations

Although the greatest sources of funding, technical support, and leadership will continue to come from donor governments, recipient governments, and UN agencies, contributions from the world of philanthropy have never been more significant. Early in the twentieth century, Rockefeller philanthropy supported efforts to eliminate hookworm, first domestically and then internationally. It has since taken on many other disease-control efforts directed toward conditions, including malaria, schistosomiasis, yellow fever, and vaccine-preventable childhood infections. In 1914, it created the China Medical Board to develop modern medicine in that country but arguably its most significant contributions to advancing global health governance were investments to establish the Johns Hopkins School of Hygiene and Public Health as well as schools of public health at Harvard and the University of Michigan. Reflecting the emergence of the new era in global health governance, in 1998 the Rockefeller Foundation established an initiative to create innovative new public-private partnerships, including the Medicines for Malaria Venture, the Global Alliance for TB Drug Development, and the International Partnership on Microbicides.[38]

Over the years, many other foundations have made important contributions to facilitating global health action, including the Ford Foundation, Atlantic Philanthropies, the Carnegie Corporation, the Bloomberg Family Foundation, the Burroughs Wellcome Trust, the Burroughs Wellcome Foundation, and the Doris Duke Charitable Foundation. The most noteworthy newcomer is the Bill and Melinda Gates Foundation. With assets of approximately $33 billion, the Gates Foundation is the largest private philanthropy in the world. Its current annual disbursements are approximately $3 billion, much of which goes to global health. Among foundations, its major commitments to GAVI (at least $1.5 billion), the Rotary International polio-eradication effort ($355 million), and the GFATM ($650 million) give it a uniquely powerful and sometimes controversial voice in global health governance. Its investments in research, implementation, and advocacy encompass enteric and diarrheal diseases; HIV/AIDS; malaria, pneumonia, tuberculosis, and neglected and other infectious diseases; family planning; nutrition; maternal, neonatal and child health; tobacco control; and vaccine-preventable diseases. Private funding now accounts for almost one-quarter of global health aid.[39]

Unlike the foundations previously mentioned, the William J. Clinton Foundation is not a grant-making organization. For nearly a decade, however, it has been a unique contributor to advancing global health. By capitalizing on the influence of former President Bill Clinton, this foundation has catalyzed many initiatives. Among these initiatives have been tremendous gains in access to HIV/AIDS treatment through negotiations with suppliers of drugs and diagnostic tests. Through successive agreements, suppliers to low-income countries have reduced the prices of first-line treatments by 50%, pediatric medicines by 90%, and second-line HIV/AIDS medicines by a cumulative reduction of 30%.[40]

CORPORATIONS AND CIVIL SOCIETY ORGANIZATIONS

Over the last decade, the corporate sector has also been making an increasing mark on global health. Although corporate initiatives are too numerous to catalog in detail, their donations of drugs are especially noteworthy. Since 1987, for example, Merck has donated ivermectin for the control of onchocerciasis (river blindness) worldwide. In 1998, in partnership with GlaxoSmithKline, this commitment was expanded to include the elimination of lymphatic filariasis; Ivermectin and GlaxoSmithKline's albendazole were coadministered in African countries and in Yemen (countries where lymphatic filariasis and onchocerciasis are coendemic). Over 21 years, more than 1 billion treatments for these infections have been provided though a large partnership.[41] Johnson and Johnson donates enough mebendazole each year to treat 25 million children for intestinal helminthes; Boehringer Ingelheim donates nevirapine to prevent mother-to-child transmission of HIV. Pfizer has proved to be a valuable and innovative partner with its support for capacity-building activities, such as the Pfizer Global Health Fellows program. Each year, this program deploys up to 50 talented employees to work on high-impact, capacity-building projects in developing countries.[42] Similarly, BD strengthens capacity through a partnership with PEPFAR to improve laboratory systems in countries highly affected by HIV/AIDS and TB.[43]

The emerging corporate role in global health is not limited to companies focused on the business of health. Companies as diverse as ExxonMobil, Warner Brothers, and Nike have engaged in important partnerships focused on controlling malaria, HIV/AIDS, and violence against girls. American Cyanamid has donated millions of dollars of the larvicide temephos to support guinea worm eradication efforts. Formal business coalitions have developed to take on issues of malaria, tuberculosis, and HIV/AIDS.[44]

The role of civil society organizations in global health predates all of those entities previously named. The WHO lists 189 NGOs with which it has an official relationship.[45] As the WHO notes:

> *No longer the domain of medical specialists, health work now involves politicians, economists, lawyers, communicators, social scientists and ordinary people everywhere. The involvement of civil society has profoundly affected not only the concepts underpinning public health but the formulation and implementation of public health programs and policies as well.*[46]

Civil society organizations span a wide array of secular and faith-based entities. They include groups with a disease-specific orientation; groups with a professional-specialty focus; charities that work on the ground; and global professional service organizations, such as Rotary International. (Rotary International is a key global partner in the WHO campaign for polio eradication.[47])

Perhaps the most exciting recent development in the United States has been the explosion in interest in global health education at universities. Suffice it to say that if governance is the constellation of mechanisms a society uses to effect collective action toward common goals, then the catalyst of the many new US multidisciplinary university programs in global health education will initiate and energize an unprecedented level of collective action.[48]

CURRENT POLICY CHALLENGES FOR INTERNATIONAL GOVERNANCE

Despite the vast inflow of resources for global health, the remaining policy challenges are significant. Perhaps today's most acute global health challenge is achieving the 3 health-related MDGs. Current trends indicate that none of these basic targets will be near achievement by 2015. Overall access to care is still lacking or suboptimal for billions of people. Access to clean water and essential medicines is uneven. Modern pharmaceuticals are often unaffordable or unavailable. Globalization has brought some health benefits to the world's poorest, but it has also fostered the transnational spread of infectious diseases, the brain drain of skilled health care workers from developing countries, and the trade in poor-quality food and pharmaceuticals. Surveillance for human and animal diseases is of variable quality and the enforcement of the relevant regulatory regimes needs improvement. Despite the challenges that remain in coordinating the many diverse players now engaged in global health, the vast increase in the commitment of both private and public wealth over the last decade is to be celebrated. Commitments have gone far beyond money and have brought forth legions of individuals who choose to commit themselves in the global context to the universal value of health. Research is steadily discovering and developing new technological interventions. New mechanisms of cooperation have been developed, and there is a growing interest in implementation science and in program evaluation to increase accountability and effectiveness. Improved global health governance to better catalyze and coordinate collective action remains an essential underpinning to meeting the diverse challenges to saving lives in all parts of the globe.

REFERENCES

1. Labisch A. Global governance in health – do historical experiences of industrialized countries teach any lessons? 2002. Available at: http://www.giga-hamburg.de/openaccess/nordsuedaktuell/2002_3/giga_nsa_2002_3_labisch.pdf. Accessed March 21, 2011.
2. Murphy FA, Nathanson N. The emergence of new virus diseases: an overview. Semin Virol 1994;5:87–102.
3. Knobler S, Mahmoud A, Lemon S, et al, editors. Learning from SARS: preparing for the next disease outbreak (workshop summary). Washington, DC: National Academies Press; 2004.
4. Relman DA, Choffnes ER, Mack A. The domestic and international impacts of the 2009-H1N1 influenza A pandemic: global challenges, global solutions (workshop summary). Washington, DC: National Academies Press; 2010.
5. Relman DA, Choffnes ER, Mack A. Infectious disease movement in a borderless world (workshop summary). Washington, DC: National Academies Press; 2010.

6. Convention on the Prohibition of the Development, Production and Stockpiling of Bacteriological (biological) and Toxin Weapons and on their Destruction. Available at: http://www.unog.ch/80256EDD006B8954/(httpAssets)/C4048678A93B6934C1257188004848D0/$file/BWC-text-English.pdf. Accessed March 21, 2011.
7. United Nations Statistics Division – Commodity Trade Statistics Database. Available at: http://comtrade.un.org. Accessed September 3, 2010.
8. Fda. Information on Adverse Event Reports and Heparin. Available at: http://www.fda.gov/Drugs/DrugSafety/PostmarketDrugSafetyInformationforPatientsandProviders/ucm112669.htm. Accessed September 21, 2010.
9. Top 15 U.S. agricultural import sources, by calendar year, $U.S. value. Available at: http://www.ers.usda.gov/Data/FATUS/DATA/McyTOP15.xls. Accessed March 21, 2011.
10. Crosse M. Drug safety: preliminary findings suggest recent FDA initiatives have potential, but do not fully address weaknesses in its foreign drug inspection program (testimony before the Subcommittee on Oversight and Investigations, Committee on Energy and Commerce, US House of Representatives). Washington, DC. The United States Government Accountability Office; 2008. (GAO-08-701T).
11. Relman DA, Hamburg MA, Choffnes ER, et al. Global climate change and extreme weather events: understanding the contributions to infectious disease emergence (workshop summary). Washington, DC: National Academies Press; 2008.
12. Kates J, Katz R. U.S. Global health policy: U.S. participation in international health treaties, commitments, partnerships, and other agreements. Menlo Park (CA): Kaiser Family Foundation; 2010.
13. Constitution of the World Health Organization. Available at: http://apps.who.int/gb/bd/PDF/bd47/EN/constitution-en.pdf. Accessed March 21, 2011.
14. The Role of the WHO in Public Health. Available at: http://www.who.int/about/role/en/index.html. Accessed March 21, 2011.
15. The WHO Agenda. Available at: http://www.who.int/about/agenda/en/index.html. Accessed March 21, 2011.
16. Gostin LO, Mok EA. Global health governance report (commissioned paper). The U.S. commitment to global health: recommendations for the public and private sectors. Washington, DC: Institute of Medicine; 2009. p. 214–8.
17. Who. Draft proposed programme budget 2010–2011. Available at: http://www.paho.org/english/gov/cd/cd48-whobpb-e.pdf. Accessed September 3, 2010.
18. The Millennium Development Goals Report 2010. New York, NY: United Nations. Available at: http://www.un.org/millenniumgoals/pdf/MDG%20Report%202010%20En%20r15%20-low%20res%2020100615%20-.pdf. Accessed September 4, 2010.
19. United Nations Declaration of Commitment on HIV/AIDS. New York: United Nations general assembly special session on HIV/AIDS. Available at: http://data.unaids.org/publications/irc-pub03/aidsdeclaration_en.pdf. Accessed March 22, 2011.
20. UNICEF 2009 Annual Report. The convention on the rights of the child. New York: UNICEF; 2009. Available at: http://www.unicef.org/publications/files/UNICEF_Annual_Report_2009_EN_061510.pdf. Accessed March 21, 2011.
21. American Veterinary Medical Association. One health initiative task force: final report. One Health - a new professional imperative. Available at: http://www.avma.org/onehealth/onehealth_final.pdf. Accessed March 22, 2011.

22. Keusch GT, Pappaioanou M, González MC, et al, editors. Sustaining global surveillance and response to emerging zoonotic diseases. Washington, DC: National Academies Press; 2009. p. 14–5.
23. WTO Agreements and Public Health: A joint study by the WHO and the WTO secretariat. Geneva (Switzerland): World Trade Organization/World Health Organization. Available at: http://www.who.int/media/homepage/who_wto_e.pdf. Accessed March 22, 2011.
24. The World Bank Annual Report 2009-Year in Review. The International bank for reconstruction and development/the world bank. Washington, DC: The World Bank; 2009. Available at: http://siteresources.worldbank.org/EXTAR2009/Resources/6223977-1252950831873/AR09_Complete.pdf. Accessed March 21, 2011.
25. Wagstaff A, Claeson M, Hecht RM, et al. Millennium development goals for health: what will it take to accelerate progress? In: Jamison DT, Breman JG, Measham AR, et al, editors. Disease control priorities in developing countries. New York: Oxford University Press and the World Bank; 2006. p. 181–94.
26. Kates J, Fischer J, Lief E. U.S. global health policy: the U.S. government's global health policy architecture: structure, programs, and funding. Menlo Park (CA): Kaiser Family Foundation; 2009.
27. Committee for the Evaluation of the President's Emergency Plan for AIDS Relief (PEPFAR) Implementation. PEPFAR implementation: progress and promise. Institute of Medicine. Washington, DC: National Academies Press; 2007.
28. Lantos T, Hyde HJ. Public Law 110–293. United States Global Leadership Against HIV/AIDS, Tuberculosis, and Malaria Reauthorization Act of 2008. H.R. 5501. Available at: http://www.govtrack.us/congress/bill.xpd?bill=h110-5501. Accessed March 22, 2011.
29. The Institute of Medicine Committee on the US Commitment to Global Health. The U.S. commitment to global health: recommendations for the public and private sectors. Washington, DC: National Academies Press; 2009. p. 137.
30. Global Health Initiative. Available at: http://www.pepfar.gov/ghi/index.htm. Accessed September 25, 2010.
31. Fallon WJ, Gayle HD. Report of the CSIS Commission on Smart Global Health Policy: a healthier, safer, and more prosperous world. Washington, DC: Center for Strategic & International Studies; 2010.
32. Board on International Health, Institute of Medicine. America's vital interest in global health: protecting our people, enhancing our economy, and advancing our international interests. Washington, DC: National Academies Press; 1997.
33. The Institute of Medicine Committee on the U.S. Commitment to Global Health. The U.S. commitment to global health: recommendations for the public and private sectors. Washington, DC: National Academies Press; 2009.
34. Lyman PN, Wittles SB. No good deed goes unpunished: the unintended consequences of Washington's HIV/AIDS programs. Foreign Aff 2010;9(4): 74–84.
35. The global fund to fight AIDS, tuberculosis, and malaria – pledges. Available at: http://www.theglobalfund.org/documents/pledges_contributions.xls. Accessed September 25, 2010.
36. About the Global Fund. Available at: http://www.theglobalfund.org/en/about/?lang=en. Accessed September 25, 2010.
37. Committee on the Economics of Antimalarial Drugs. Saving lives: buying time: economics of malaria drugs in an age of resistance. Washington, DC: National Academies Press; 2004.

38. Rockefeller Foundation- Our History. Available at: http://www.rockefellerfoundation.org/who-we-are/our-history. Accessed September 25, 2010.
39. Bloom DE. Governing global health. Finance Dev 2007;44(4). Available at: http://www.imf.org/external/pubs/ft/fandd/2007/12/bloom.htm. Accessed September 13, 2010.
40. Clinton Health Access Initiative. Available at: http://www.clintonfoundation.org/what-we-do/clinton-health-access-initiative. Accessed September 25, 2010.
41. Mectizan Donation Program. Available at: http://www.mectizan.org/pdci. Accessed September 12, 2010.
42. Global Health Fellows: Pfizer Investments in Health. Available at: https://globalhealthfellows.pfizer.com/login.asp?ReturnUrl=home.asp. Accessed September 12, 2010.
43. BD (Becton, Dickinson and Company): BD's Global Health Initiative. Available at: http://www.bd.com/globalhealth/initiative/assistance.asp. Accessed September 12, 2010.
44. Global Business Coalition on HIV/AIDS, Tuberculosis and Malaria. Available at: http://www.gbcimpact.org/. Accessed September 25, 2010.
45. World Health Organization. List of NGOs in official relations with WHO. Available at: http://www.who.int/civilsociety/relations/official_relations/en/. Accessed September 12, 2010.
46. World Health Organization. Civil Society Initiative (CSI). Available at: http://www.who.int/civilsociety/health/en/. Accessed March 21, 2011.
47. Rotary International/The Rotary Foundation. Available at: http://www.rotary.org/en/SERVICEANDFELLOWSHIP/POLIO/Pages/ridefault.aspx. Accessed September 25, 2010.
48. Merson MH, Page KC. The dramatic expansion of university engagement in global health: implications for US policy: a report of the CSIS Global Health Policy Center. Washington, DC: Center for Strategic & International Studies; 2009.

The Role of Treaties, Agreements, Conventions, and Other International Instruments in Global Health

Jennifer Kates, MA, MPA[a,*], Rebecca Katz, PhD, MPH[b]

KEYWORDS

- International agreements • Treaties • International law
- Global health multilateral agreements

International agreements, commitments, and partnerships are an integral part of every nation's global health engagement. As nations become more reliant on each other for cohesive development of global health policies and practice, and globalization increasingly makes health challenges in one part of the world concerns for all nations, the importance and use of international agreements in framing policy and national commitments have increased.[1,2] These agreements establish political and legal commitments, formalize international relationships, and coordinate roles and responsibilities in an increasingly complex and interconnected world. Some of these agreements are legally binding under international law, and may also be binding under national law, whereas others are non-binding but may confer political, diplomatic, governance, or other expectations on parties.[1,2]

Whether a nation chooses to become party to an agreement may send an important signal to the international community regarding national priorities, help to shape the dialog on key global health issues, and may in turn serve to influence the direction of national policies and programs. Despite the importance of these agreements, no single database is currently available for cataloguing the range of international agreements pertaining to health.

The authors have nothing to disclose.
[a] Global Health & HIV Policy, Kaiser Family Foundation, 1330 G Street, NW, Washington, DC 20005, USA
[b] Department of Health Policy, The George Washington University, School of Public Health and Health Services, 2021 K Street, NW, Suite 800, Washington, DC 20006, USA
* Corresponding author.
E-mail address: jkates@kff.org

Infect Dis Clin N Am 25 (2011) 455–475
doi:10.1016/j.idc.2011.02.002 id.theclinics.com
0891-5520/11/$ – see front matter

To better understand the scope and content of international health agreements, and the status of country participation, the authors reviewed international agreements that are currently in place, looking specifically at multilateral instruments or partnerships—those in which three or more parties,[3] including governmental membership, are involved—to identify those that either directly focus on or encompass health. The authors identified 50 of these agreements, including those that are legally binding under international law and those that are non-binding. This article defines the different types of agreements, describes the process through which governments enter into these agreements, evaluates the legality of agreements under international law, and assesses participation by member states.

METHODOLOGY

To compile the list of international agreements on health, multiple databases, reports, and other sources were reviewed, including the United Nations Treaty Collection, which provides a database of all multilateral treaties, including full text and status, deposited with the United Nations (UN), as all nations are obligated to do under the UN charter.[4] The U.S. Department of State's required annual report to Congress on all *Treaties in Force*,[5] the U.S. Library of Congress reference collection on Treaties,[6] and other reference documents and databases were also reviewed.[1,7] Each agreement was reviewed to assess its scope, purpose, and content, and only those that were health-specific or had a significant health component and were currently active were included in the final analysis. In addition, only multilateral international agreements were included; bilateral (country-to-country) agreements were not included, although nations are party to thousands of these agreements. Although the authors endeavored to identify agreements that met these criteria, selection involved some level of subjective judgment.

BACKGROUND

History

Governmental involvement in international health activities began more than a century ago, motivated by both public health and economic concerns as nations increasingly sought to promote international trade and travel while also protecting their countries from external disease threats by regulating shipping ports and other border access points.[8] Largely to support international trade and shipping, in 1851 France convened the first International Sanitary Conference to begin standardizing international quarantine regulations and practices and to develop an international system of disease notification. Subsequent conferences ensued, and in 1892, participating nations approved the first standardized set of health measures—The International Sanitary Convention.[8–12] Although this convention marked the first international health agreement of its kind,[13] few multilateral agreements generally, let alone on health specifically, existed until after World War II, when several interrelated factors led to their growing use, including rising globalization and transborder movement; increasing international cooperation connected to foreign policy agendas, particularly in the post–Cold War period; the need to address new and complex areas internationally (eg, new disease threats and environmental challenges, as most recently evidenced by H1N1 in 2009); and the rise in the number of sovereign states, which makes the use of multilateral agreements not only more necessary but also more efficient compared with each nation negotiating individually with a large and growing number of unique states.[1,2,14,15]

In 1907, the global community established the first international health office, the "Office International d'Hygiène Publique," located in Paris, to oversee international health agreements.[12] The duties of this office were transferred to the World Health Organization (WHO) after its creation in 1948. Some international health agreements continue to be overseen and, in several cases, administered by the WHO, whereas others are tied to different UN entities, non-UN bodies, and independent governing boards.

TAXONOMY OF INTERNATIONAL AGREEMENTS

The term *international agreement* is broad and used to capture a range of different instruments and arrangements between countries or organizations of states, including multilateral agreements (those between three or more nations or bodies) and bilateral agreements (those between two nations). Agreements can also occur between a state and an organization or between organizations. Agreements are generally in written form, and may be either legally binding or carry no weight of legal force.[16] According to the UN, the degree of formality chosen for an international agreement depends partly on the particular problem or issue to be addressed and the political implications for and intent of the parties.[17]

Under international law, an international agreement is considered to be legally binding if it conveys the intention of its parties to create legally binding relationships under international law and has entered into force, or become active. However, because the term *agreement* may be used to encompass, and even formally name, all types of international instruments, the official name of an agreement may not always be indicative of its legality, formality, or strength, and may instead reflect political or other factors.[2,18,19] These different types of agreements are described in the following sections.

Legally Binding Agreements

Treaties

The strongest legally binding agreement, whether multilateral or between two nations, is a treaty. According to the Vienna Convention on the Law of Treaties 1969, a treaty is an international agreement "governed by international law, whether embodied in a single instrument or in two or more related instruments and whatever its particular designation."[20] It is a compact between at least two nations or between nations and an international organization, carrying with it international legal obligations that are binding under international law.[21] Although no international rule specifies when the term *treaty* should be used to formally name an international instrument, it is, according to the UN, "employed for instruments of some gravity and solemnity."[3] Nations become parties to treaties through ratifying or acceding to them, a process described in more detail in a later section. Once ratified, treaties establish international legal obligations and may also create domestic legal obligations on members.

However entry into a treaty can be qualified through submission of Reservations, Understandings and Declarations (also known as *RUDS*), which serve to modify or clarify the meaning of the agreement.[1,3] For example, when the United States agreed to the International Health Regulations in 2005, a legally binding agreement that provides a framework for coordinating the detection, reporting, and international response to events that may constitute a public health emergency of international concern (PHEIC), it did so with a reservation stating that the United States would assume the obligations of the agreement to the extent possible, given the federalist system of government, and three understandings relating to different aspects of the International Health Regulations.[22] Likewise, India submitted a reservation indicating that it would consider yellow fever to constitute a PHEIC and how it will classify infected areas. Five other nations (China, Greece, Portugal, Tonga, and Turkey) submitted understandings, clarifying both specific sections of the regulations and interpreting other nations' reservations, and one nation (Iran) submitted an objection to the reservation and understandings submitted by the United States.

Protocols

A protocol amends or otherwise supplements an existing treaty, including addressing issues of interpretation, establishing additional rights or obligations, or implementing components of a treaty. Numerous types of protocols exist, as defined by the UN, including protocols of signature, optional protocols, protocols based on a framework treaty, protocols to amend an agreement, and protocols as supplementary treaty.[19] Although additional or supplementary to an existing treaty, all protocols require ratification by member nations, which in most countries will entail the same process as treaty ratification.

Non-Binding Agreements

In addition to legally binding agreements, many other types of international agreements and partnerships may carry other obligations or expectations (eg, political, financial) although not legally binding under international law.[1,2] Non-binding agreements may include commitments to organizations or common goals, and may have various names (eg, declarations, principles, communiqués). The formal name of an agreement, which may be chosen for political reasons, does not always match its technical definition.[21] The most common names and arrangements used for non-binding agreements are described in the following sections (however, these terms can be used to apply to legally binding agreements in some cases, and therefore each agreement must be evaluated separately).

Commitments to UN organizations, programs, funds, or specialized UN agencies

In addition to legally binding agreements for which the sole purpose is to establish a UN organization (eg, the WHO), others similarly establish UN organizations or specialized UN agencies (eg, the Joint United Nations Programme on HIV/AIDS) but are not legally binding under international law. Instead, they confer some other kind of commitment (eg, political, financial, governance, membership) to the organization. Once these organizations have been established, they often promulgate regulations and procedures applicable to the subject matter covered by the organization. Typically, through choosing to become a member of an international organization, nations agree to allow the organization to propose technical regulations and procedures that set priorities, identify collective action, provide a regulatory framework, and mobilize resources.[23] Membership in the organization, however, does not mandate that each nation follows the regulations and procedures, but these often become standards for global guidance.

Declarations, principles, and other international agreements/partnerships

A *declaration* is a term that can be applied to various international agreements, and is generally applied to those that are non-binding. In fact, the term *declaration* is often chosen for agreements in which parties declare shared intentions, but have no binding obligations.[19] In the context of multilateral agreements, declarations are often made by an international institution such as the UN. For example, the United Nations' Declaration of Commitment on HIV/AIDS[24] is designed to guide and foster commitment and support by governments to address HIV/AIDS but does not legally bind them to do so.

Similarly, statements of principle are not legally binding, yet mark a commitment to a set of ideas, norms, and challenges. For example, 192 countries are committed to the principles outlined by the UN Millennium Development Goals (MDGs),[25] which, set for 2015, represent an agreed on set of goals to promote poverty reduction, education, maternal health, and gender equality, and to combat child mortality, HIV, and other diseases. In addition, principles may eventually form the core of future international agreements, including those that are legally binding.

Some international agreements and partnerships also involve multiple nations in which a UN organization serves as Secretariat, coordinator, fiduciary agent, or advisor, or in which multiple nations are involved in the governing body. Nations may make legally binding commitments to the partnership (often in terms of resources), but the partnership itself is not binding under international law, and a legal contract between the nation and the organization is not necessarily required. For example, although 14 donor country governments (plus the European Union) partner, sit on the board of, and provide funding to the Global Alliance for Vaccines and Immunisations[26]—a global health public and private partnership designed to accelerate access to vaccines and stimulate development of new immunization technology—this partnership does not bind nations to fund, engage in, or support these endeavors under international law.

Because these types of agreements and partnerships are not legally binding on nations, their power and impact are variable. In some cases, they may not result in any action or change. In other instances, they may serve to mobilize nations to do more and help forge a global agenda,[27] as in the case of the Global Polio Eradication Initiative, launched by the WHO in 1988, which mobilized nations around the global goal of eradicating polio; or the MDGs, which have mobilized nations around eight international development goals and is shaping the global agenda around development aid.[28]

NATIONAL CONSIDERATION OF INTERNATIONAL AGREEMENTS

National engagement in international agreements is multifaceted, and may include promoting the development of an international agreement on a particular issue, participating in the drafting of an agreement, negotiating on its terms, and ultimately deciding whether to become a party. A decision to participate in negotiating an international agreement, let alone becoming party to it, is shaped by many factors, including national policy priorities, security concerns, economic interests, health and humanitarian concerns, leveraging potential, and the formality and legality of the agreement, including its obligations on parties.[1,2] An international agreement forged with other nations may be the result of a single government or subset of governments' policy priority, wherein one or several nations actively engages the international community to produce an agreement around an issue of interest. It may also arise in the absence of a prior national interest but subsequently lead to or otherwise impact government policies.

The strongest international instruments are those that are legally binding under international law, although non-binding international agreements may be politically binding or otherwise establish certain obligations between parties, and may carry "significant moral and political weight."[2] In some cases, a non-binding agreement may be seen as more flexible and easier to pursue than legally binding agreements, while still providing an opportunity to achieve policy goals. Regardless, once an agreement is "on the books" and a country has made an official decision to either be a party to it or not, this at the very least signals a national position and may impact national, regional, or global policy on that issue.

The process of becoming party to an international agreement is guided by the 1969 Vienna Convention on the Law of Treaties. Ratification, also known as *acceptance*, *approval*, or *accession*, is defined by the Convention as "the international act so named whereby a State establishes on the international plane its consent to be bound by a treaty."[20] Although the ratification process varies by nation, it generally involves Parliamentary (or Congressional) approval and may necessitate the adoption of domestic legislation to execute the terms of the treaty within a particular country.[20] Treaties "enter into force" (ie, become legally binding under international law) only after a specified number of parties ratify (or accede to) the treaty.[21] **Table 1** provides an overview of the international treaty process.

In most countries, the authority to negotiate, conclude, sign, and ratify a treaty is outlined in its constitution, and often involves both the executive and legislation branches of government (**Table 2**). The negotiation, conclusion, and signature process is usually controlled by the head of state (as in Australia, the United States, the United Kingdom, and throughout the European Union), and the ratification process rests with the legislative branch. The legislative branch is also involved when implementing legislation is required to execute a treaty.

Still, the process varies somewhat by nation. In the United States, for example, both the executive and legislative branches of government are involved in the international agreement process, although their roles vary depending on the type of agreement (**Fig. 1**).[1,2,19] Although the power to negotiate and enter into legally binding and other international agreements rests with the US Executive Branch (primarily at the Department of State), Congress plays an important oversight and approval role for some types of legally binding agreements to enable them to enter into force and, for any international treaty to be considered a treaty under United States law, two-thirds of the Senate must give its "advice and consent."[29] At the same time, the United States may also become a party to an international treaty through "Executive Agreement," which does not always involve Congress. In the United Kingdom, the executive (Prime Minster or Foreign Secretary) negotiates and signs treaties, except for certain European Union treaties, which are signed by the Queen. Unlike the United States and most other nations, parliamentary approval of treaties is not required, although in practice, several mechanisms have been established that allow oversight and scrutiny by Parliament.[30] Even when Parliamentary or Congressional approval is required, countries may have different thresholds, with the United States requiring two-thirds of the Senate to approve treaty ratification, whereas other nations, such as France and South Africa, require a simple majority of both houses of their legislatures.

FINDINGS

Based on a review of current multilateral agreements, 50 were identified that either directly focused on or encompassed health (see Appendix 1 for detailed list of agreements). These are most likely to be treaties or protocols to treaties (n = 26), followed by declarations, principles, or other types of agreements (n = 18) (**Table 3**). Of the 50 agreements, 26 are legally binding under international law. The 50 agreements span many topics and issues, and can be categorized into several broad areas. They are most likely to address specific diseases such as HIV, tuberculosis, polio, or malaria (n = 11), followed by those that address health through an environmental

Table 1
Overview of treaty process

Procedural Step for Treaty	Process
Negotiation	Each nation authorizes an individual to participate in negotiating the text of an agreement on behalf of the country.
Conclusion	Conclusion of a treaty marks the end of negotiation. This term is never fully defined by the Vienna Convention, but usually means either the treaty is open for signature or, in some cases, entry into force.
Acceptance or approval	The Vienna Convention allows for consenting states to express "acceptance" or "approval" of a treaty, provided that the agreement allows this action. This action expresses the consent of the state to be bound by a treaty. This practice is used be certain states instead of ratification, when national (domestic) constitutional law does not require a treaty to be ratified by the head of state.
Signature	A designated representative of a nation signs the treaty. This act is meant to express the willingness of the nation to continue the treaty-making process, and qualifies the country to proceed to ratification, acceptance of approval. Once a nation has signed the treaty, it becomes a "signatory" to the agreement, although this does not yet formally bind the nation to the agreement.
Ratification (or Accession or Act of Formal Confirmation)	Ratification is when a nation indicates its consent to be bound to a treaty. The host government goes through internal processes to approve the treaty and, if necessary, enact legislation to give domestic effect to the treaty, and then formally notifies the depository of the treaty. After ratification, and once the treaty enters into force, a nation becomes a "party" to the agreement. Accession is when a nation decides to become a party to the treaty after it has already been negotiated, signed, ratified, and entered into force by other states. It has the same effect as ratification and the nation goes through the same internal process for domestic approval. An Act of Formal Confirmation is also the same as ratification, but is the term used for international organizations that express consent to be bound by a treaty.
Reservations, Understandings, or Declarations	At the time of acceptance, approval, signature, ratification or accessing, nations can enter reservations, understandings, or declarations (known as RUDS) to the agreements. RUDS are submitted by a nation to exclude or alter the effect of certain parts of an agreement to the country, or clarify how the country interprets certain provisions.

Data from The United Nations Treaty Collection. Available at: http://treaties.un.org/. Accessed September 1, 2010; and Aust A. Modern treaty law and practice. 2nd edition. Cambridge (New York): Cambridge University Press; 2007.

Table 2
Treaty ratification: role of executive and legislative branches in select countries

Country	Executive	Legislature/Parliament
Brazil	President: negotiates and signs	Congressional approval required: absolute majority in both houses (Chamber of Deputies and the Federal Senate)
France	President: negotiates and signs	Parliamentary approval required: simple majority in both chambers (National Assembly and Senate)
South Africa	President: negotiates and signs	Parliamentary approval required: simple majority in both houses (National Assembly and National Council of Provinces)
United States	President: negotiates and signs	Congressional approval required: two-thirds majority in Senate. The executive branch, however, can use the constitutional powers of the president to enter into agreements (thus called "Executive Agreements") without or with only limited congressional involvement. These agreements hold the same weight as other treaties under domestic law.
United Kingdom	Prime Minster or Foreign Secretary, signs; certain European Union treaties are signed by the Queen	Parliamentary approval not required/no formal role of parliament (there are exceptions and Ponsby Rule)

Data from Refs.[1,29–36]

lens (n = 7) or as a trade/intellectual property issue (n = 6). A smaller number address health for specific populations, such as women, children, and refugees, through a human rights framework (n = 5), as part of security/preparedness (n = 4), or within agreements focused on water/sanitation (n = 3) or food/nutrition (n = 3) (**Table 4**).

The remainder are generally international health agreements to establish or support organizations that address health issues, such as the WHO, the directing and coordinating authority for health within the UN system; the World Bank, the world's major international financing organization that focuses on poverty reduction efforts in low and middle-income countries, including through health projects; and the International Finance Facility for Immunisation, an innovative financing organization that raises funds for immunization by issuing bonds in capital markets. The remainder may also be agreements that address multiple health issues across a range of areas.

Participation in these international agreements varies. Of the 26 legally binding treaties and protocols, 10 have universal or near-universal membership (defined as 95% of all member states; there are 192 member states in the United Nations and 193 in the WHO). In these cases, the countries that have not become party to the agreement denote a policy position, as in the case of the Convention on the

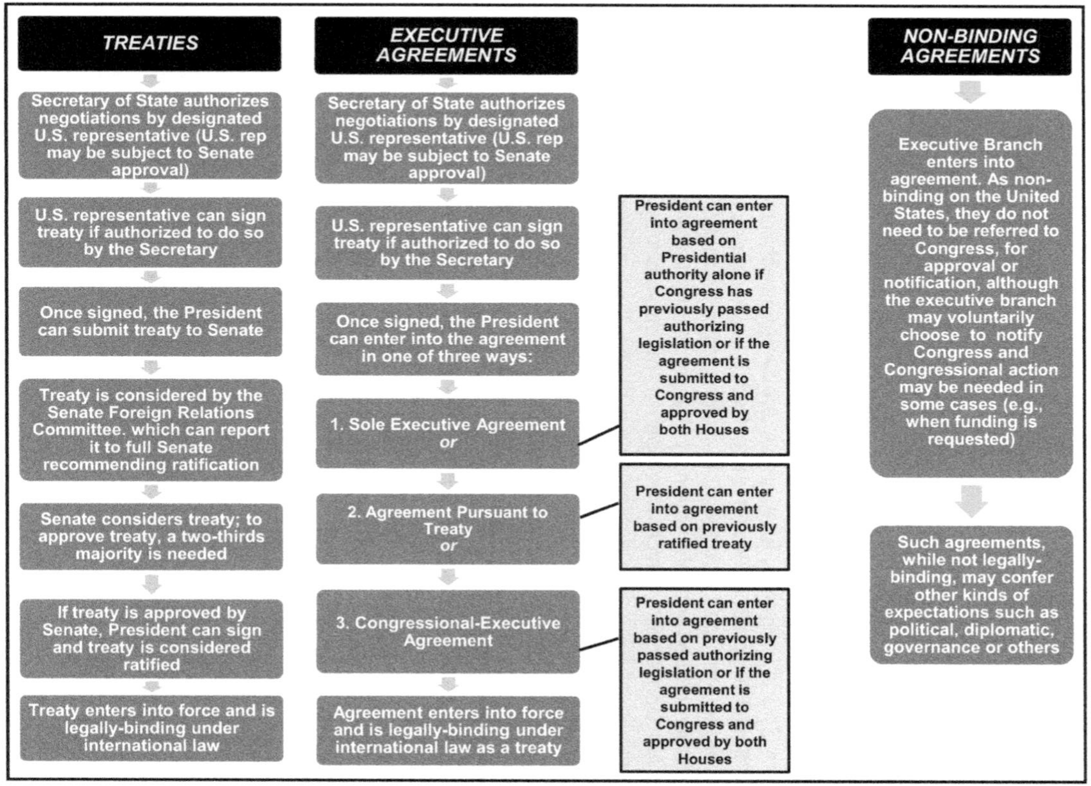

Fig. 1. How the US Government becomes a party to an international agreement. (*From* Kates J, Katz R. U.S. Participation in International Health Treaties, Commitments, Partnerships, and Other Agreements. Menlo Park, CA: Kaiser Family Foundation; 2010. Available at: http://www.kff.org/globalhealth/8099.cfm. Accessed March 20, 2011; with permission.)

Table 3
Number of international agreements on health according to type of agreement

Type	Number
Treaties	21
Protocols	5
Commitment to UN organization, program, fund, or specialized agency	6
Declarations, principles, and other international agreements/partnerships	18
International total	50

Elimination of All Forms of Discrimination Against Women, in which only seven countries (the United States, Sudan, Somalia, Iran, Nauru, Palau, and Tonga) have not ratified, and the Convention on the Rights of the Child, in which only the United States and Somalia have not ratified.

The other 16 legally binding agreements have less membership because of various other factors. Four agreements, for example, are designed either to focus membership within a particular region (the Pan American Health Organization, Pan American Sanitary Code for the Americas, and the Convention on the Protection and Use of Transboundary Watercourses and International Lakes) or to target a particular set of nations (the Food Aid Convention, which was open to membership by a subset of donor governments). In addition, four agreements with less than universal membership are Word Trade Organization treaties, each of which has economic implications related to international trade issues.

Among the remainder are several others that have ideological or political differences or for which the issue is not seen as a high priority for or relevant to some countries, such as the Biological and Toxin Weapons Convention and the Stockholm Convention on Persistent Organic Pollutants. Two legally binding agreements with less than universal membership focus on specific populations, including people with disabilities and refugees. One agreement, which is open for signature and ratification, has yet to receive the minimum number of required parties to enter into force. **Table 5** provides an overview of legally binding international health agreements according to year and membership.

Table 4
International agreements on health according to focus of agreement

Focus	Number	Legally Binding
Disease	11	0
Environment	7	7
Trade/intellectual property	6	6
Population-specific	5	4
Health security/preparedness	4	2
Water	3	2
Food/nutrition	3	1
Other	11	4
International total	50	26

Table 5
Legally binding international health agreements according to year and membership

Name of Agreement	Year of Entry Into Force	Members/Parties to Agreement	Non-Parties
Treaties			
Biological and Toxin Weapons Convention (BWC)	1975	163 parties	13 additional countries have signed but not yet become a party to the agreement
Convention on Biological Diversity (CBD)	1993	193 parties	Two non-state parties: the United States and Somalia
Convention on the Elimination of All Forms of Discrimination Against Women (CEDAW)	1981	186 parties	Countries that are not a party to the agreement include the United States, Sudan, Somalia, Iran, Nauru, Palau, and Tonga
Convention on the Law of Non-Navigational Uses of International Watercourses	Not yet entered into force (too few nations signed/ratified agreement)	19 parties	Most countries have not signed or ratified this agreement
Convention on the Protection and Use of Transboundary Watercourses and International Lakes (Water Convention)	1996	37 parties	Most European nations are party to the agreement
Convention on the Rights of the Child (CRC)	1990	193 parties	Only the United States and Somalia are not party to the agreement
Convention on the Rights of Persons with Disabilities	2008	95 parties	An additional 52 countries have signed but not yet become a party to the Convention
Food Aid Convention (1999)	1999	25 parties	Donors included in the Convention are Argentina, Australia, Canada, the European community and its member states, Japan, Norway, Switzerland, and the United States
Pan American Health Organization (PAHO)/ Pan American Sanitary Code	1924	35 parties	Includes all countries in the Americas

(*continued on next page*)

Table 5
(continued)

Name of Agreement	Year of Entry Into Force	Members/Parties to Agreement	Non-Parties
Stockholm Convention on Persistent Organic Pollutants (POPs)	2004	171 parties	14 States have signed but not yet become parties to the Convention
United Nations Framework Convention on Climate Change	1994	194 parties	All states are party
Vienna Convention for the Protection of the Ozone Layer	1988	196 parties	All states are party
World Health Organization (WHO)	1948	193 parties	All states are party
World Intellectual Property Organization (WIPO)	1970	184 parties	Non-parties include Solomon Islands, Marshall Islands, Micronesia, Nauru, Palau, Timor-Leste, Tuvalu, and Vanuatu
World Health Organization Framework Convention on Tobacco Control (FCTC)	2005	169 parties	14 additional countries have signed the agreement but have not yet become a party to it
World Trade Organization– General Agreement on Trade in Services (GATS)	1995	153 parties	31 additional countries have observer status but have not yet become a party to the agreement
World Bank	1945	Membership in each institution IBRD: 187 IDA: 170 IFC: 182 MIGA: 175 ICSID: 144	The following countries are not members of the World Bank IBRD: Andorra, Cuba, North Korea, Liechtenstein, Monaco, Nauru, and Tuvalu
World Health Organization Revised International Health Regulations (IHR, 2005)	2007	194 parties	All states are party

World Trade Organization–Agreement on the Application of Sanitary and Phytosanitary Measures (WTO-SPS)	1995	153 parties	31 additional countries have observer status but have not yet become a party to the agreement
World Trade Organization– Agreement on Technical Barriers to Trade (WTO-TBT)	1995	153 parties	31 additional countries have observer status but have not yet become a party to the agreement
World Trade Organization–Trade-Related Aspects of Intellectual Property Rights (WTO-TRIPS)	1995	153 parties	31 additional countries have observer status but have not yet become a party to the agreement
Protocols			
Cartagena Protocol on Biosafety to the United Nations Convention on Biological Diversity	2003	160 parties	11 countries have signed but not yet become a party to the Protocol
Kyoto Protocol to the United Nations Framework Convention on Climate Change	2005	192 parties	All parties to the UN Framework Convention on Climate Change are parties, except the United States, Afghanistan, and Somalia
London Protocol on Water and Health to the Convention on the Protection and Use of Transboundary Watercourses and International Lakes	2005	24 parties	An additional 14 countries have signed but not yet become a party to the Protocol
Montreal Protocol on Substances that Deplete the Ozone Layer to the Vienna Convention for the Protection of the Ozone Layer	1989	196 parties	All states are party
Protocol to the United Nations Convention Relating to the Status of Refugees (1967)	1967	144 parties	Non-parties include most of South and Southeast Asia and the Middle East

Abbreviations: IBRD, International Bank for Reconstruction and Development; ICSID, International Centre for Settlement of Investment Disputes; IDA, International Development Association; IFC, International Finance Corporation; MIGA, Multilateral Investment Guarantee Agency.

In addition to these legally binding agreements are many non-binding agreements, which represent other kinds of commitments by nations. Among the non–legally binding commitments to UN organizations, programs, funds, or specialized agencies, there is almost universal membership in the Food and Agriculture Organization, the United Nations Children's Fund, and the United Nations Development Program, and a majority membership in the United Nations Population Fund. Among declarations, principles, and other international agreements, some of the UN-driven global declarations and initiatives, such as the Millennium Development Goals and United Nations General Assembly Special Session, have almost universal endorsement. Other initiatives focus on countries able to provide funding to support a particular endeavor, such the Global Fund to Fight AIDS, Tuberculosis and Malaria, separating out donor and recipient member states. Other partnerships target countries based on geography or shared borders, such as the North America Leaders' Summit.

DISCUSSION

There are numerous health-related international agreements that nations participate in, providing an important component of global health engagement. This review identified 50 international agreements that focus on or encompass health, including approximately half that are legally binding under international law. Although many have universal or near-universal participation by nations, others have fewer members, reflecting a range of political, economic, and other factors. The identified agreements span many topics and areas, with most addressing specific diseases, such as HIV, reflective of the large-scale disease-specific initiatives that have arisen over the past decade. Several others address health through an environmental lens or as a trade/intellectual property issue, two areas for which international attention and cooperation are increasingly seen as needed. A smaller number address health for specific populations, such as women, children, and refugees, through a human rights framework, as part of security/preparedness, or within agreements focused on water/sanitation or food/nutrition, although at least some of these areas, such as security/preparedness and food/nutrition, have risen on the international agenda more recently.

Given rising globalization and increasing international cooperation and complexity, as evidenced by the recent international mobilization to respond to H1N1, the use of multilateral agreements in the realm of health probably will continue to grow. Although these agreements do not currently dominate many nations' global health engagement, they do represent a less-known but important area of consideration in any assessment of global health policy. This involvement helps to not only define governmental roles in global health but also shape the international agenda on key global health issues, and sends a signal to the international community about current and future priorities. Moving forward, it will be important to continue to monitor international health agreements, and studies such as those described can help to inform an increasingly complex and interconnected global health response.

ACKNOWLEDGMENTS

This work is based on a report by Kates and Katz, U.S. Participation in International Health Treaties, Commitments, Partnerships, and Other Agreements. Menlo Park: Kaiser Family Foundation. Report #8099. September 2010. Available at: http://www.kff.org/globalhealth/upload/8099.pdf. The authors would also like to acknowledge the assistance of Sarah Elrod in preparing this document.

APPENDIX 1: DETAILED LIST OF AGREEMENTS BY TYPE, LEGAL STATUS, AND FOCUS

Name of Agreement (N = 50)	Type of Agreement	Legally Binding Under International Law (N = 26)	Focus Area
Biological and Toxin Weapons Convention (BWC)	Treaty	Yes	Health security: biologic weapons
Cartagena Protocol on Biosafety to the Convention on Biological Diversity	Protocol	Yes	Environment: biosafety; modified organisms
Convention on Biological Diversity (CBD)	Treaty	Yes	Environment: biodiversity
Convention on the Elimination of All Forms of Discrimination Against Women (CEDAW)	Treaty	Yes	Population: women
Convention on the Law of Non-Navigational Uses of International Watercourses	Treaty	No	Water
Convention on the Protection and Use of Transboundary Watercourses and International Lakes (Water Convention)	Treaty	Yes	Water
Convention on the Rights of the Child (CRC)	Treaty	Yes	Population: children
Convention on the Rights of Persons with Disabilities	Treaty	Yes	Population: persons with disabilities
Doha Declaration on the TRIPS Agreement and Public Health	Other international agreement/ partnership	Yes	Trade/intellectual property
Food Aid Convention (FAC)	Treaty	Yes	Food/nutrition
Food and Agriculture Organization (FAO)	Commitment to UN organization, program, fund, or specialized UN agency	No	Food/nutrition

(*continued on next page*)

APPENDIX 1 (*continued*)

Name of Agreement (N = 50)	Type of Agreement	Legally Binding Under International Law (N = 26)	Focus Area
Global Alliance for Vaccines and Immunisation (GAVI)	Other international agreement/ partnership	No	Disease: vaccines and immunizations
Global Fund to Fight AIDS, Tuberculosis and Malaria (Global Fund)	Other international agreement/ partnership	No	Disease: HIV/AIDS, tuberculosis, and malaria
Global Health Security Initiative	Other international agreement/ partnership	No	Health security: public health preparedness
Global Polio Eradication Initiative	Other international agreement/ partnership	No	Disease: polio
Group of Eight Health Commitments	Other international agreement/ partnership	No	Multiple issues
International Conference on Population Development (ICPD) Programme of Action	Other international agreement/ partnership	No	Health and development
International Finance Facility for Immunisation (IFFIm)	Other international agreement/ partnership	No	Disease: vaccines and immunizations
International Health Partnership (IHP+)	Other international agreement/ partnership	No	Health partnerships; health systems strengthening
International Partnership on Avian and Pandemic Influenza	Other international agreement/ partnership	No	Disease: avian and pandemic influenza
Kyoto Protocol to the United Nations Framework Convention on Climate Change	Protocol	Yes	Environment: greenhouse gasses
London Protocol on Water and Health to the Convention on the Protection and Use of Transboundary Watercourses and International Lakes	Protocol	Yes	Water

(*continued on next page*)

APPENDIX 1 (*continued*)

Name of Agreement (N = 50)	Type of Agreement	Legally Binding Under International Law (N = 26)	Focus Area
Millennium Development Goals (MDGs)	Other international agreement/ partnership	No	Multiple issues
Montreal Protocol on Substances that Deplete the Ozone Layer to the Vienna Convention for the Protection of the Ozone Layer	Protocol	Yes	Environment: greenhouse gasses
North America Leaders' Summit (Formally the Security and Prosperity Partnership of North America)	Other international agreement/ partnership	No	Health security: public health preparedness
Pan American Health Organization (PAHO)/Pan American Sanitary Code	Treaty	Yes	International health organization
Paris Declaration on Aid Effectiveness	Other international agreement/ partnership	No	Financing/ international aid
Protocol to the United Nations Convention Relating to the Status of Refugees (1967)	Protocol	Yes	Population: refugees
Roll Back Malaria (RBM)	Other international agreement/ partnership	No	Disease: malaria
Stockholm Convention on Persistent Organic Pollutants (POPs)	Treaty	Yes	Environment: pollutants
Stop TB Partnership	Other international agreement/ partnership	No	Disease: tuberculosis
Joint United Nations Programme on HIV/AIDS (UNAIDS)	Commitment to UN organization, program, fund, or specialized UN agency	No	Disease: HIV/AIDS

(*continued on next page*)

APPENDIX 1 (*continued*)

Name of Agreement (N = 50)	Type of Agreement	Legally Binding Under International Law (N = 26)	Focus Area
Three Ones Principles	Other international agreement/ partnership	No	Disease: HIV/AIDS
UNITAID	Other international agreement/ partnership	No	Disease: HIV/AIDS, tuberculosis, and malaria
United Nations Children's Fund (UNICEF)	Commitment to UN organization, program, fund, or specialized UN agency	No	Population: children
United Nations Development Programme (UNDP)	Commitment to UN organization, program, fund, or specialized UN agency	No	Health and development organization
United Nations Framework Convention on Climate Change	Treaty	Yes	Environment: greenhouse gasses
United Nations General Assembly Special Session (UNGASS): Declaration of Commitment to HIV/AIDS	Other international agreement/ partnership	No	Disease: HIV/AIDS
United Nations Population Fund (UNFPA)	Commitment to UN organization, program, fund, or specialized UN agency	No	Health and development organization
United Nations World Food Programme (WFP)	Commitment to UN organization, program, fund, or specialized UN agency	No	Food/nutrition
Vienna Convention for the Protection of the Ozone Layer	Treaty	Yes	Environment: greenhouse gasses
WHO Framework Convention on Tobacco Control (WHO FCTC)	Treaty	Yes	Tobacco
World Bank	Treaty	Yes	Financing/ international aid

(*continued on next page*)

APPENDIX 1 (*continued*)

Name of Agreement (N = 50)	Type of Agreement	Legally Binding Under International Law (N = 26)	Focus Area
World Health Organization (WHO)	Treaty	Yes	International health organization
World Health Organization Revised International Health Regulations (IHR, 2005)	Treaty	Yes	Health security: public health preparedness
World Intellectual Property Organization (WIPO)	Treaty	Yes	Trade/intellectual property
World Trade Organization–Agreement on the Application of Sanitary and Phytosanitary Measures (WTO-SPS)	Treaty	Yes	Trade/intellectual property
World Trade Organization–Agreement on Technical Barriers to Trade (WTO-TBT)	Treaty	Yes	Trade/intellectual property
World Trade Organization–General Agreement on Trade in Services (GATS)	Treaty	Yes	Trade/intellectual property
World Trade Organization–Trade Related Aspects of Intellectual Property Rights (WTO-TRIPS)	Treaty	Yes	Trade/intellectual property

REFERENCES

1. Congressional Research Service. A study prepared for the Committee on Foreign Relations, United States Senate. Treaties and other international agreements: the role of the United States Senate. Washington, DC: Government Printing Office; 2001.

2. Congressional Research Service. International law and agreements: their effect upon U.S. law. RL32528. Washington, DC: Government Printing Office; 2010.
3. United Nations. Treaty handbook. United Nations Treaty Collection. Available at: http://treaties.un.org/doc/source/publications/THB/English.pdf. Accessed March 18, 2011.
4. The United Nations Treaty Collection. Available at: http://treaties.un.org/. Accessed September 1, 2010.
5. US Department of State. Treaties in force. Available at: http://www.state.gov/s/l/treaty/tif/index.htm. Accessed August 1, 2010.
6. The Library of Congress. Treaties. The Library of Congress Web site. Available at: www.thomas.gov/home/treaties/treaties.html. Accessed September 1, 2010.
7. University of California Berkeley. Reference guide: treaties and international agreements. Doe & Moffitt Libraries' Web site. Available at: http://www.lib.berkeley.edu/doemoff/govinfo/intl/gov_trtygde.html. Accessed March 20, 2011.
8. International Sanitary Conference. Proceedings of the international sanitary conference: provided for by joint resolution of the Senate and House of Representatives in the early part of 1881. Washington, DC: Government Printing Office; 1881.
9. Huber V. The unification of the globe by disease? The international sanitary conferences on Cholera, 1851–1894. Hist J 2006;49:453–76.
10. Harvard University, International Sanitary Conferences. Contagion: historical views of diseases and epidemics. Harvard University Library Open Collections Program Web site. Available at: http://ocp.hul.harvard.edu/contagion/sanitaryconferences.html. Accessed August 1, 2010.
11. Howard-Jones N. The Scientific background of the international sanitary conferences 1851–1938. Geneva (Switzerland): World Health Organization; 1975.
12. Protocoles de la Conférence Sanitaire Internationale. Ouverte à Paris le 9 avril 1859. Rome (Italy): Impr. Nationale de J. Bertero; 1892.
13. Howard-Jones N. The Pan American Health Organization: origins and evolution. Geneva (Switzerland): World Health Organization; 1981. Available at: http://whqlibdoc.who.int/iph/WHO_IPH_5.pdf. Accessed March 18, 2011.
14. Fidler DP. The challenges of global health governance. New York: Council on Foreign Relations Press; 2010. Available at: http://www.cfr.org/publication/18985/global_governance_monitor.html#/Public%20Health/Overview%20Video/. Accessed March 20, 2011.
15. Council on Foreign Relations. Issue brief: the global health regime. Council on foreign relations, global governance monitor: public health. Available at: http://www.cfr.org/publication/18985/global_governance_monitor.html#/Public%20Health/Overview%20Video/. Accessed March 20, 2011.
16. Garner BA, editor. Black's law dictionary. 8th edition. Eagan (MN): Thomson West; 2004.
17. Definition of key terms used in the UN treaty collection. United Nations treaty collection. Available at: http://treaties.un.org/Pages/Overview.aspx?path=overview/definition/page1_en.xml. Accessed March 18, 2011.
18. Congressional Research Service. International agreements on climate change: selected legal questions. R41175. Washington, DC: Government Printing Office; 2010.
19. United Nations. Treaty reference guide. United Nations treaty collection. Available at: http://untreaty.un.org/ola-internet/Assistance/Guide.htm. Accessed August 1, 2010.

20. Vienna convention on the law of treaties. Vienna (Austria): United Nations; 1969. Available at: http://untreaty.un.org/ilc/texts/instruments/english/conventions/1_1_1969.pdf. Accessed March 20, 2011.
21. Aust A. Modern treaty law and practice. 2nd edition. Cambridge (MA): Cambridge University Press; 2007.
22. World Health Organization. International Health Regulations (2005). Appendix 2: reservations and other state party communications in connection with the international health regulations (2005). 2nd edition. Geneva (Switzerland): World Health Organization; 2008.
23. World Health Organization. Constitution of the World Health Organization. World Health Organization website. Available at: http://www.who.int/governance/eb/who_constitution_en.pdf. Accessed March 20, 2011.
24. United Nations. Declaration of commitment on HIV/AIDS: "Global Crisis—Global Action." United Nations web site. Available at: http://www.un.org/ga/aids/coverage/FinalDeclarationHIVAIDS.html. Accessed March 18, 2011.
25. United Nations. Millennium development goals. United Nations website. Available at: http://www.un.org/millenniumgoals/. Accessed March 18, 2011.
26. GAVI alliance web site. Available at: http://www.gavialliance.org/. Accessed March 18, 2011.
27. Landry MD, Raman S. Millennium development goals (MDGs): a global policy paradox. World Health Popul 2007;9(3):5–8.
28. History of polio. The global polio eradication initiative web site. Available at: http://www.polioeradication.org/. Accessed September 1, 2010.
29. Government of the United States. 1 U.S.C. 112a; 1 U.S.C. 112b; 1 U.S.C. 113. Available at: www.state.gov/s/l/treaty/authorities/domestic/65799.htm. Accessed March 18, 2011.
30. United Kingdom House of Parliament. Factsheet P14: procedure series, treaties. London: House of Commons. Available at: http://www.parliament.uk/factsheets. Accessed March 20, 2011.
31. U.S. Department of State. Information from the office of the assistant legal adviser for treaty affairs website. Available at: http://www.state.gov/s/l/treaty/index.htm. Accessed March 20, 2011.
32. U.S. Department of State. Foreign affairs manual, 11 FAM 700, treaties and other international agreements. Available at: http://www.state.gov/m/a/dir/regs/fam/c23019.htm. Accessed March 20, 2011.
33. Government of Brazil. Constitution of Brazil, title IV, chapter 1, section 1. Available at: http://www.v-brazil.com/government/laws/titleIV.html. Accessed March 20, 2011.
34. Government of France. Constitution of France, title IV. Available at: http://www.assemblee-nationale.fr/english/8ab.asp#VI. Accessed March 20, 2011.
35. Government of South Africa. Constitution of South Africa. Chapter 14, section 231. Available at: http://www.info.gov.za/documents/constitution/1996/96cons14.htm. Accessed March 20, 2011.
36. United Kingdom. Foreign & commonwealth office, treaties, practices and procedures. Available at: http://www.fco.gov.uk/en/publications-and-documents/treaties/practice-procedures/full-powers. Accessed February 12, 2011.

Index

Note: Page numbers of article titles are in **boldface** type.

Infect Dis Clin N Am 25 (2011) 477–483
doi:10.1016/S0891-5520(11)00027-4 id.theclinics.com
0891-5520/11/$ – see front matter

D

E

G

T

U

W